# Implementing Outcome-Based Home Care: A Workbook of OBQI, Care Pathways and Disease Management

Melinda Huffman, RN, MSN, CCNS
Director of Nursing Education
Motlow State Community College
Tullahoma, Tennessee

**JONES AND BARTLETT PUBLISHERS**
*Sudbury, Massachusetts*
BOSTON   TORONTO   LONDON   SINGAPORE

*World Headquarters*
Jones and Bartlett Publishers
40 Tall Pine Drive
Sudbury, MA 01776
978-443-5000
info@jbpub.com
www.jbpub.com

Jones and Bartlett Publishers
Canada
2406 Nikanna Road
Mississauga, ON L5C 2W6
CANADA

Jones and Bartlett Publishers
International
Barb House, Barb Mews
London W6 7PA
UK

*Production Credits*
Acquisitions Editor: Kevin Sullivan
Production Manager: Amy Rose
Editorial Assistant: Amy Sibley
Production Assistant: Tracey Chapman
Marketing Manager: Ed McKenna
Manufacturing Buyer: Amy Bacus
Composition: Bill Noss Graphic Design
Cover Design: Kristin Ohlin
Printing and Binding: Courier Stoughton
Cover Printing: Courier Stoughton

Printed in the United States of America
08 07 06 05 04 10 9 8 7 6 5 4 3 2 1

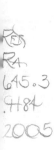

# Table of Contents

# Guidelines for Use

## WORKBOOK LAYOUT

The material is presented in a workbook format, designed to enhance learning through an active, self-instructional process. It is divided into five major chapters, with sub-sections in each chapter. The chapter material progresses from basic to advanced. Information in each section is likewise arranged, with information in one section preparing the user for the one to follow. Each section is prefaced with learning objectives, agency-specific data and resources needed to complete the applications within the section, and core terms and concepts that are discussed within the section.

You are encouraged to assemble the agency-specific data and resources prior to beginning each chapter.

The body of each section begins with an *Introduction of the topic*, including *Definitions*. *Patient Examples* are given throughout, ending with basic and/or advanced *Concept Applications* and *Agency Applications* of the material. *Concept Applications* are designed to help the user understand the subject matter by providing examples of the concepts learned. *Agency Applications* are designed to guide the user through actual application of the concepts to his or her agency's patient population(s). Some agency applications direct you to use a certain form located in the Appendices. These forms are placed here collectively so that additional copies can be easily made for the application, as well as for future agency use.

As you complete each agency application, a critical component of your agency's action plan is being written for the implementation of outcome-based patient care. Upon completion of the workbook, the action plan should likewise be at or near its completion. For this reason, the workbook's maximum impact can be realized when all members of the agency's leadership team take part in its applications.

Throughout the workbook, *Guiding Questions* are presented to stimulate critical reasoning, to prompt further questions, and to raise issues particular to the agency's patient population and processes of care delivery.

A *Reference List* is provided at the end of each section. The *Appendices* include an Internet resource listing for best practices, action plans for performance activities in OBQI, care pathway development and implementation, and disease management. A *Subject Index* concludes the workbook.

## APPLICATION OF MATERIAL

An agency need not feel that it must implement OBQI, care pathways, *and* disease management in order to achieve success with implementing outcome-based patient care; quite the contrary. Agencies whose primary focus is only OBQI/OBQM are encouraged to use this material to better understand its concepts and as a reference for applying these concepts into everyday practice through performance improvement.

Care pathways can be used as a perfect vehicle for implementing standards of care and outcomes measurement for both OBQI and disease management. The use of care pathways is the agency's decision to make, but one that is highly recommended. The workbook guides you through the development of a care pathway, which can also be used to help evaluate your own existing pathways or to evaluate new ones for purchase.

You are encouraged to finish all of the workbook material and applications should you decide to launch a disease management initiative. Disease management can be used to augment service lines, to further refine the care provided for specific patient populations and/or to enter into alliances with hospitals as part of a continuum of care. It is outcome-based patient care in an advanced form.

## CHAPTER SUMMARIES

*Chapter 1* covers basic outcomes terminology, the use and application of outcomes measurement and standards of care, variance, and variance management. It describes the critical link between outcomes achieved and standards that are implemented, a factor often misunderstood and frequently omitted in the development of outcome-based systems of care.

This chapter also discusses patient compliance and its effect on outcomes achieved. The terms *Adherence* and *Concordance* are new terms beginning to surface in the literature in place of *compliance*. However, compliance is used in this text, as it continues to be the term most often used in current literature and the one most familiar to healthcare professionals.

*Chapter 2* serves multiple purposes:

- It helps the agency establish its focus for outcome-based patient care by guiding the user through applications that identify the agency's primary patient population(s) and that ascertain staff competency and expertise relative to these patient groups.
- It extrapolates critical principles from the OBQI manual and presents them in quick reference format, so users can readily access and apply this information to OASIS outcome examples throughout the workbook. It also provides simple, easy-to-understand applications of OBQI concepts.
- It directs the use of the user agency's OASIS outcome reports for analysis based on results of this workbook's applications.
- It can be used for OBQI orientation for new management level staff.
- It outlines the necessary steps in the development and implementation of care pathways and describes essential components of initiating disease management in home care.
- It discusses the importance of patient compliance in outcomes management, and how to measure compliance outcome indicators.

*Chapter 3* explains how to use agency desired outcomes to formulate the staff competency assessment and performance appraisal. Enhanced accountability exists when agency standards of care and accurate measurement of outcomes are implemented.

*Chapter 4* discusses how interventions selected to achieve specific outcomes warrant a financial analysis of cost versus benefit to patients and to the agency. This chapter provides a framework and rationale for the application of financial outcomes data.

*Chapter 5* demonstrates how to analyze outcomes from a marketing perspective, how to base marketing strategies on outcomes achieved, how to affect physician practice patterns, and how to prepare outcome presentations for customers.

# Acknowledgments

Several individuals gave me a tremendous amount of encouragement and support while this workbook was written.

An untold amount of gratitude goes to *Colleen Miller*, a special colleague and true friend, who contributed the chapters of *Finance* and *Marketing and Business Development*, and whose professional capability and personal convictions I truly admire and respect. Colleen has many years of clinical, administrative, and healthcare outcomes management experience, including a role as a corporate senior vice-president with responsibility for homecare disease management. Her contribution was invaluable. Our countless hours of preparation and collaboration on this project made the journey exhausting at times and comical too, but most of all worthwhile and an incredible experience.

Immense appreciation goes to *Carolyn Humphrey, Editor, Home Healthcare Nurse*, my mentor and special friend. Without her guidance and direction, this project would have made it to the attic long before it ever made it to publication. She continues to be my rock, and I will be forever grateful to her for believing in me.

A special thanks to *Annette Lester*, a very best friend and professional colleague, who continued to encourage me by affirming, "Home care needs this so badly." This kept me determined to complete the project.

Sincere thanks to the librarians at the University of Alabama, Birmingham, AL, the University of the South, Sewanee, TN, and Motlow State Community College, Tullahoma, TN, who were especially helpful in assisting me to access hundreds and hundreds of articles for the review of the literature.

Finally, and most importantly, much gratitude and appreciation go to my husband, *Oren* and son, *Wes*, and *Mother* and *Dad*, who always allowed me to pursue my professional goals by placing no obstacles in my path and by being a wonderful and loving Christian family. And to my Jack Russell Terrier, my constant companion through it all.

— *Melinda H. Huffman*

# Foreword

*In particular, providers must accept responsibility and
accountability for patient outcomes that occur
over episodes of care for which payment is received.
In sum, the prospective payment system has ushered in
not only a new era of financing home health care
under Medicare, but also a new era of accountability.*

Shaughnessy, P., Crisler, K., Hille, D., Schlenker, R. (2002)

From the Summary of the Report on OASIS and Outcome-Based Quality
Improvement in Home Health Care: Research and Demonstration Findings,
Policy Implications and Considerations for Future Change.

# Introduction

As payers have demanded to know what the worth of home care is relative to other healthcare settings, the need for measuring actual results (outcomes) of care has become a priority. Homecare providers are in a new *outcomes* environment. This environment emphasizes accountability and responsibility for managing care quality based on outcomes achieved. We must evaluate these outcomes against national benchmarks, as well as the agency's own prior results. We must not only be able to demonstrate the results of the patient care we provide, but also be able to enhance the quality of care based on these results.

This workbook and reference is designed for home managers, leadership staff, senior clinicians and administrators, performance improvement (PI) and staff development coordinators, and instructors of community and home health nursing, as well as point-of-care software companies that develop outcome-based pathways for homecare patients.

It provides the information and tools necessary to implement outcome-based home care using OASIS and agency supplemental outcomes, Outcome-Based Quality Improvement/Outcome-Based Quality Monitoring (OBQI/OBQM), best practice, care pathways, and disease management. Additionally it helps users learn how to integrate outcomes into the agency's marketing and business strategies, financial decisions, and staff competency and performance appraisals.

The Manager and Director, who have little time to extract and organize information from multiple sources to implement this new approach, will find the workbook helpful in:

- Presenting outcomes terminology and concepts in the context of familiar, everyday patient examples
- Outlining "have-to-know" OBQI/OBQM information in a succinct, step-by-step format
- Providing applications for direct, real-time agency use
- Developing outcome-based performance appraisals that enhance staff accountability for implementation of agency standards

The Homecare Executive will find information for:

- The consideration of disease management as a vehicle through which hospital and home alliances may be formed
- Correlating clinical and financial outcomes data
- Discovering how patient outcomes can potentially affect physician practice patterns and decisions of managed care organizations
- Preparing outcome presentations for customers

PI and Staff Development Coordinators can use the information for:

- Orienting new leadership staff to outcome-based care and OBQI/OBQM
- Teaching the principles of outcome-based care
- Preparing staff presentations
- Developing agency standards of care
- Writing meaningful, supplemental agency outcomes
- Aggregating and trending agency supplemental outcomes data
- Developing care pathways that address the needs of the agency's patient populations
- Conducting competency in OBQI/OBQM

Nursing Instructors will find it particularly useful when:

- Teaching outcome-based terminology and concepts
- Teaching students how to evaluate patient care and response in the home setting based on outcomes achieved
- Explaining how outcomes are affected by various clinical interventions and patient compliance

Software companies that provide applications for point-of-care devices will have the critical link for successfully:

- Developing pathway standards of care according to clinical practice guidelines
- Writing outcomes that correspond with the implementation of standards of care
- Aggregating and trending outcomes data
- Incorporating patient teaching as a standard of care
- Enhancing the efficiency of their application's design

Upon completion of the workbook, the user will have the knowledge and skills necessary to:

1. Define terms and apply core concepts essential to the implementation of outcome-based home care.
2. Develop agency standards of care and supplemental outcomes according to best practices.
3. Analyze OBQI/OBQM outcome reports and implement performance improvement initiatives accordingly.
4. Develop best-practice care pathways that are relevant to the agency's patient population(s) and evaluate existing ones for effectiveness or purchase.
5. Develop a homecare disease management initiative as part of a healthcare continuum.
6. Aggregate and trend agency supplemental outcomes data.
7. Integrate agency outcomes data into:
   - Clinical practice and patient teaching materials
   - Staff competency and performance evaluations
   - Finance applications
   - Marketing and business development
8. Quantify agency success through the implementation of outcome-based home care.

# The Foundation of Outcome-Based Home Care: Outcomes Measurement and Standards of Care

## Outcomes and Outcomes Measurement

### LEARNING OBJECTIVES

Upon completion of this topic, you will be able to:

1. Describe basic outcomes terminology.
2. Explain the difference between outcomes and goals.
3. Identify different types of outcomes.
4. Describe how outcomes are selected for measurement.
5. Explain how outcomes are measured.
6. Describe appropriate timeframes for outcomes measurement.
7. Write acceptable and appropriate outcome indicators.
8. Determine accuracy of outcomes data.
9. Describe the importance of reliability and validity of outcome indicators.
10. Describe the benefits of benchmarking outcomes data.

### AGENCY-SPECIFIC DATA/RESOURCES NEEDED

N/A

---

**CORE TERMS AND CONCEPTS**

- Outcome
- Outcome-based patient care
- Outcomes management
- Outcomes measurement
- Outcome indicator(s)
- Outcome percent
- Outcome report
- Supplemental outcomes
- OASIS outcomes
- Accuracy of outcomes data
- Validity
- Reliability
- Internal & External Benchmarking

# INTRODUCTION

Hill (1999) describes *outcome-based patient care* as an approach that uses patient outcome measurements as the basis for the provision of patient care. In this context, outcomes, or the results of care rendered, serve as the *starting point for improving care quality*. In other words, the quality of care you deliver, expressed as a measurement, is used as the basis for improving it.

This same premise is used in the Outcome-Based Quality Improvement (OBQI) initiative (Shaughnessy, Crisler, and Schlenker, 1997) of the Centers for Medicare and Medicaid Services (CMS). It is also used in the development of agency care pathways and best practices that incorporate the use of patient outcomes to improve quality of care. Outcomes are also used by clinicians and patients alike to make more informed healthcare decisions (Outcomes Research, 2000).

Outcome-based patient care entails the use of *outcomes management*, the ongoing measurement of outcomes and their correlation with treatment (Epstein and Sherwood, 1996). Outcomes management includes the development, design, measuring, reporting, tracking, and revision of healthcare outcomes (Peters, Cowley, and Standiford, 1999; Whittington, 1998).

This section explains basic outcomes terminology, concepts, and outcomes measurement, analyzes the differences among various types of outcomes, examines the importance of data accuracy, and discusses external and internal benchmarking of outcomes data.

## WHAT IS A HEALTHCARE OUTCOME?

While an *outcome* is most often defined as the result of care rendered (Jennings, Staggers, and Brosch, 1999), the end-result of care (Camann, 2001), or responses, behaviors, and feelings of care provided (Kleinpell, 2003), CMS (2002b), defines an outcome as the change in patient health status between two or more time points, which may be due to the care provided or to the natural progression of illness. An outcome is not a process, nor a plan of care, nor an assessment, nor a goal.

## THE DIFFERENCE BETWEEN A GOAL AND AN OUTCOME

A *goal* is what one desires to attain (Merriam-Webster, 2002); an *outcome* is the result that is attained. For example, a physician asks the patient to weigh daily and record the weight for one week. The patient's goal is to weigh daily for seven days and enter the weights on a calendar. However, at the end of seven days, the patient forgot to weigh on two of the days. The *goal* was seven days; the *outcome* was five days of seven.

Another example is the goal of a spouse to be able to administer an injection to the patient within six visits. The spouse is able to administer the injection in four visits. The *goal* was within six visits; the *outcome* was four visits.

To better understand the difference, first think of a desired goal in the form of a statement that can be measured. For example, you have a patient with a new diagnosis of diabetes. One *goal* is that the patient/caretaker will verbalize signs and symptoms of hypo/hyperglycemia by the third visit. However, the patient and caretaker verbalized signs and symptoms of hypo/hyperglycemia by the fourth visit. This example shows that the *goal* was not met. A measurement of the *outcome* indicated that the *goal* was met by the fourth visit, not the third as intended.

**1**A

## CONCEPT APPLICATION:
### Differentiating Between Goals and Outcomes

In each example below, differentiate between the statements that reflect a desired *goal* and an end-result *outcome*.

*Example 1*

- The patient/caretaker will independently use a glucometer by visit five.

  _____

- The patient independently used a glucometer by visit six. _____

*Example 2*

- The patient/caretaker verbalized components of a low fat, low cholesterol diet

  prior to discharge. _____

- The patient/caretaker will verbalize the components of a low fat, low choles-

  terol diet prior to discharge. _____

*Answers: Example 1—goal, outcome; Example 2—outcome, goal*
*Rationale: A goal states what is to be attained; an outcome states what is attained.*

## GOALS, OUTCOMES, AND THE 485 (POC)

In preparing a plan of care (CMS 485), clinicians are to develop *measurable* goals with the patient/caretaker, outlining what is to be accomplished, when, and by whom (Humphrey and Milone-Nuzzo, 1996). When a goal is appropriately written, an end-result outcome is implied and can be measured. Some examples of goals with implied end-result outcomes that are appropriate for the 485 include:

- Patient or caretaker will demonstrate proper dressing change for wound by visit eight.
- Patient will achieve "X" score on the Functional Independence Measure (FIM) within 60 days.
- Patient/caretaker will be compliant with maintaining an accurate, daily blood glucose log throughout the length of service.

---

### CONCEPT APPLICATION:
### Writing Goals for Outcome Measurement

Using the previous examples for guidance, write a simple goal appropriate for outcome measurement for the patient who has a pressure ulcer.

_____

_____

_____

*Answer: (example) Patient/caretaker will independently change the wound dressing within 10 visits.*

Write a simple goal appropriate for outcome measurement for the patient who is receiving oxygen.

_____

_____

_____

*Answer: (example) Patient/caretaker will verbalize five safety measures of managing oxygen use and equipment.*

---

## TYPES OF HEALTHCARE OUTCOMES

There are many ways to group similar outcomes. Let's review some of these categories and study respective examples. Peters, Cowley, and Standiford (1999) categorize the following groups of outcomes as those most frequently used as quality indicators of care:

- Clinical
- Functional
- Medical
- Financial
- Customer Satisfaction

Kleinpell (2003) discusses two additional types of outcomes suitable for measurement:

- Compliance
- Knowledge

CMS (2002b) further categorizes OASIS outcomes into three groups for use in OBQI and Outcome-Based Quality Monitoring (OBQM). These three groups include some of the types listed previously. These are:

- End-Result Outcomes
- Utilization Outcomes
- Adverse Events Outcomes

## Clinical

Clinical outcomes may be described as results that are measured in physiological parameters, describing the status of a health condition (Jennings, Staggers, and Brosch, 1999).

Examples include: **vital signs, level of dyspnea, stage of pressure ulcer, level of pain or anxiety, diagnostic values, and occurrence of infection**.

List two additional types of *clinical* outcomes:

1._____

2._____

**1**A

## Functional

Functional outcomes are those that measure the patient's level of physical functioning (Arslanian, 2001) and return to activities of daily living (Peters, Cowley, and Standiford, 1999).

Examples include: **range of motion, strength, and independence with activity, and may be expressed in ambulation distance, and in degrees of movement as evidenced through functional measurement scales**.

List two additional types of *functional* outcomes:

1._____

2._____

## Medical

Medical outcomes relate to procedures performed, medical treatment regimens, and complications of treatment or implanted devices (Johlin, 1999).

Examples include: **mortality rates, morbidity rates, procedure complication rates, re-admission rates, and return to ER.**

List two additional types of *medical* outcomes:

1._____

2._____

## Financial

Financial outcomes indirectly measure the appropriate utilization of resources and procedures (Peters, Cowley, and Standiford, 1999) and are generally compared to baseline data.

Examples include: **average cost per patient per episode, average episodes per diagnosis, average HHRG reimbursement per episode, and average supply costs.**

List two additional types of *financial* outcomes:

1._____

2._____

*Customer Satisfaction*

Satisfaction outcomes indicate the level at which expectations are met (Arslanian, 2001).

Examples include: **timeliness of returned phone calls, satisfaction with pain control, and satisfaction with treatment.** *Quality of life* is also becoming an outcome of interest (Jennings, Staggers, and Brosch, 1999).

List two additional types of *satisfaction* outcomes:

1._____

2._____

*Compliance*

Patient compliance is the degree to which the patient follows health interventions as agreed with the healthcare provider (Cleemput and Kestlefoot, 2002; Cramer, 2002).

Examples include: **compliance with medication regimen, with home exercise program, with special diet, and with obtaining and recording periodic weights.** Compliance outcomes may be expressed in statements that include who is compliant within a specific timeframe, such as "patient is compliant with ADA diet while on service."

List two additional types of *compliance* outcomes:

1._____

2._____

*Knowledge*

Because patient and caretaker education is the number one intervention in the provision of home care (Waggoner, 1999), knowledge acquired by the patient and/or caretaker during service must be measured.

Positive knowledge outcomes enhance clinical outcomes by providing the patient with the information and understanding necessary to provide better self-care, increase compliance with treatment regimens, and enhance health and wellness practices (Lamb-Harvard, 1997).

Examples include: **verbalization or description of treatment regimen, verbalization of adverse signs and symptoms, verbalization of medication dose and side effects, demonstration of glucometer, and demonstration of injection**. Knowledge (educational) outcomes are also reflected in statements that include who is to acquire the knowledge within a specific timeframe, such as "patient independently demonstrates use of glucometer by visit four."

List two additional types of *knowledge* outcomes:

1._____

2._____

## OASIS OUTCOMES

OASIS outcomes are reported for OBQI and OBQM. OBQI uses *end-result* outcomes and *utilization* outcomes as a basis for improving care quality, while OBQM uses *adverse event* outcomes.

## End-Result Outcomes

OBQI combines physiological, functional, cognitive, behavioral, and emotional outcomes into a single category called *End-Result* or *Health Status Outcomes* (CMS, 2002b). These are further divided into two types:

1. *Improvement Outcomes*—A patient improves if he or she is less severely ill, disabled, or dependent at discharge than at the start of care (or resumption of care) (CMS, 2002b).
   Examples of improvement outcomes are expressed as **Improvement in ambulation, Improvement in toileting, Improvement in dyspnea, and Improvement in incontinence**.
2. *Stabilization Outcomes*—A patient has stabilized if he or she is no more disabled/dependent (not worsened) at discharge than at the start of care (CMS, 2002b).
   Examples of stabilization outcomes are expressed as **Stabilization in bathing, Stabilization in dyspnea, and Stabilization in transferring**.

## Utilization Outcomes

These outcomes are obtained from the use of health services or discharge information (CMS, 2002b).
Examples include **Hospital admission, Use of emergent care, and Discharge to the community**.

## Adverse Event Outcomes

The term adverse event is used to specify an unusual or *undesired* patient occurrence that happens during the course of care (CMS, 2002b).
Examples include: **Emergent care due to fall or injury, Substantial decline in health status, Emergent care due to wound deterioration/infection, and Development of urinary tract infection**.

## OUTCOME INDICATORS

An outcome indicator or outcome measure is a parameter that is assessed or evaluated to reflect the quality of an intervention or service (Kleinpell, 2003; Merboth and Barnason, 2000). *An outcome indicator is evaluated or measured to determine the outcome.* According to this definition, a properly written goal can be considered an outcome indicator.

Outcomes are not all expressed in the same manner. For example, while a financial outcome may be expressed as the average HHRG reimbursement, an Outcome Assessment and Information Set (OASIS) outcome is expressed as *Improvement in bathing.* By the same token, not all outcome measures or indicators are written the same. Look closely at the following examples of outcome measurement tools and note the differences in the way the outcome indicators are written and measured.

*Example 1 – OASIS*
In OASIS/OBQI (CMS, 2002b), the outcome of *Improvement in Dsypnea* is partly generated by clinicians entering the following patient responses on OASIS item *M0490: When is the patient dyspneic or noticeably short of breath?*

0 – Never, patient is not short of breath
1 – When walking more than 20 feet, climbing stairs
2 – With moderate exertion (while dressing, using commode or bedpan, walking distances more than 20 feet)

3 – With minimal exertion (while eating, talking, or performing other activities of daily living or with agitation)

4 – At rest (day and night)

*Example 2 – Iowa Outcomes Project: Nursing Outcomes Classification (NOC)*

Moorehead, Johnson, and Maas (2004) express outcome measures as indicators. These outcome indicators cover a myriad of subject areas; many are appropriate for home care.

One area is **Knowledge: Diet**.

Definition used by clinicians: *Extent of understanding conveyed about recommended diet.*

Outcome indicators: (excerpt only)

• Description of rationale for diet
• Description of foods allowed in diet
• Description of strategies to change dietary habits

Measurements used for this indicator related to the extent of understanding are: 1=none; 2=limited; 3=moderate; 4=substantial; 5=extensive

*Example 3 – Care Pathways*

Outcome measures or outcome indicators seen in many care pathways are written as goals ("Critical pathways—an acute," 1994). Some examples are:

1. Patient is compliant with exercise program while on service.
2. Patient/caretaker verbalizes adverse signs and symptoms to report to physician/nurse by visit two.
3. Patient/caretaker demonstrates proper care of a colostomy by visit ten.

The outcome is measured by the clinician as met, not met, or not applicable at the time, and is written by the agency. Sidorov (2003) recommends keeping measures or indicators simple and useful.

## SELECTING OUTCOME INDICATORS FOR MEASUREMENT

Outcome indicators selected for measurement should clearly reflect the changes expected to occur in response to the intervention (Strickland, 1997). For example, look at the following outcome indicator: *Patient/caretaker demonstrates proper subcutaneous injection technique by the end of visit five.*

The intervention appropriate to achieve this outcome includes educating the patient and/or caretaker how to read the markings on the syringe, draw up the medication, prepare the skin, insert the needle, pull back the plunger, inject medication, withdraw the syringe and needle, and properly dispose them. There is a clear relationship between the nursing intervention and the outcome expected.

Let's look at several ways that outcome indicators are selected for measurement.

### 1) Federal Mandate

CMS mandates the use of OASIS by all Medicare/Medicaid certified agencies to generate and use outcomes to improve care quality (Crisler, Baillie, and Conway, 2003). CMS has selected a number of specific outcome indicators for this purpose. For example, OASIS data set items *MO450: Current number of pressure ulcers at each stage* and *MO830/840: Emergent care for wound infections, deteriorating wound status* generate OASIS outcomes that are expressed as:

*Increase in number of pressure ulcers* and
*Emergent care for wound infections, deteriorating wound status*

## 2) Agency Choice

In addition to OASIS-mandated outcomes, an agency may select or write its own supplemental outcome indicators based on primary patient population, patient and procedure volume, quality of care issues, cost-effectiveness, adverse events, and/or agency standards of care. These outcome indicators (measures) may come from a variety of sources, such as professional expertise, national associations or organizations, research findings, published texts, and performance improvement (PI) initiatives.

For example, because diabetes is a high volume, high-cost diagnosis to manage, patient and caretaker education has emerged as a critical component of the care provided (Renders, Valk, Griffin, Wagner, Van Eijk, and Asssendleft, 2001). An agency writes its outcome indicators (goals) related to patient/caretaker knowledge that the American Diabetic Association (ADA) recommends for patient self-care management (Mensing, Boucher, Cypress, Weinger, Mulcahy, Barta et al., 2003). The agency delineates its time frames for outcome measurement. It uses the ADA-published information as the foundation for writing its outcome indicators. These outcome indicators include:

- Patient/caretaker independently demonstrates the use of a glucometer by visit five.
- Patient/caretaker verbalizes signs and symptoms of hypo/hyperglycemia by visit three.
- Patient/caretaker demonstrates proper foot care by the end of week four.
- Patient/caretaker verbalizes sick day guidelines by visit ten.
- Patient's finger stick glucose will be within physician-selected parameters by discharge.

In another example, an agency provides vascular infusion services to a large adult population with a wide range of diagnoses. Agency managers decide to measure the following outcome indicator for these patients:

*No phlebitis or infection at the vascular access insertion site while on service.*

The agency measures this outcome at discharge for all patients with vascular infusion devices.

## 3) Companies That Warehouse and Aggregate Outcomes Data

Some companies warehouse outcomes data for agency member use. Agencies pay a fee to become clients. These companies aggregate outcomes data for the purpose of agency comparison, including state or regional level data. Outcomes data may stem from OASIS software, agency financial analyses, staffing, and productivity. Outcomes data are typically generated via agency participation in periodic surveys and OASIS outcomes. The company designs the survey that is completed by agency members and/or provides OASIS data according to geographic location and clinical interest, as requested by provider members.

## 4) Disease Management Continuum

Homecare agencies have increasing opportunities to become part of a disease management continuum of care. As agencies become actively involved, we will be asked to continue the measurement of outcomes that begin in acute care. While this approach is collaborative, outcomes that affect acute care are likely to have already been selected for continued measurement by homecare providers.

## 5) Purchased Care Pathways

Care pathways that already have outcomes designed within the format can be purchased from an outside source. When you select the pathway, you have in essence selected the outcomes for measurement. For example, a pathway designed to guide the care for a patient with a fracture may include these outcome indicators:

- Patient/caretaker verbalizes components of a neurological/circulatory assessment by visit two.
- Patient/caretaker demonstrates neurological/circulatory assessment by visit three.
- Patient/caretaker describes why elevation of affected part and proper alignment are essential by visit three.

The outcomes in purchased care pathways must have relevance to the agency's patient populations.

## 6) Managed Care Organizations (MCOs)

Many MCO disease management programs incorporate outcome indicators that the MCO wants to measure for its covered patient populations. If your agency has a contract with an MCO, it is prudent that you be knowledgeable of outcomes it deems important and consider measuring these as appropriate to the MCO's patient groups. Medical directors of MCOs can be very helpful in recommending outcome measures related to their covered patient populations.

For example, your agency provides care for a large number of physical rehabilitation patients through a contract with an MCO. Because of the large volume of patients cared for, your agency meets at least annually with the MCO's medical director. As a result of a discussion, the agency decides to measure outcomes related to the *level of patient independence at discharge*.

## OUTCOME MEASUREMENT

*Outcome measurement* is a process of observing, describing, and quantifying indicators of outcomes (Blancett and Flarey, 1998). It is the action the clinician takes to determine patient status or other indicators relative to the outcome in question. For example, when a clinician documents a response to an OASIS item, he or she is observing or measuring the patient's status at that time. In another example, an agency writes the outcome indicator: *Patient/caretaker will demonstrate proper injection technique by visit seven.* A clinician quantifies or measures the outcome when he or she determines that the patient/caretaker can or cannot administer the injection.

Ideally, a baseline measurement and an end measurement are made to determine what the outcome is. For example, the OASIS outcome: *Increase in the number of pressure ulcers*, is quantified or measured via the OASIS software calculation of the number of pressure ulcers on admission versus the number at discharge or transfer (CMS, 2002b).

In another example, an agency measures an outcome relative to the occurrence of constipation in patients whose mobility is impaired and who are taking pain medication daily. The goal (outcome indicator) is: *Patient will have a bowel movement at least every three days while on service.* On admission, the clinician asks the patient for the date of his or her last bowel movement and begins measuring the outcome every three days from this point forward.

In a third example of a new diabetic, an agency measures the outcome indicator: *Patient/caretaker will demonstrate independent use of glucometer by visit five.* Prior to teaching, the clinician makes a simple measurement of whether the individual can independently use a glucometer. This is followed by another measurement at or before visit five.

In a fourth example, agencies incorporating outcome indicators from the Nursing Outcomes Classification (NOC) (Moorehead, Johnson, and Maas, 2004) measure outcomes through the use of a *Likert* scale. For example, one NOC outcome indicator measures the patient's *Extent of understanding when describing the potential for food and medication interaction.* The following scale is used to measure the patient's or caretaker's response of this particular outcome:

1=none
2=limited description
3=moderate description
4=substantial description
5=extensive description

The clinician *measures the outcome* when he or she selects the number that best represents the extent of understanding that the patient/caretaker has.

1A

---

### CONCEPT APPLICATION:
### Identifying Measurable Outcome Indicators

Identify the items below that represent the measurement of an outcome indicator.

☐ 1. Clinician evaluates OASIS M0420 (Frequency of pain)—on admission, follow-up, and discharge. Evaluations result in a patient outcome.

☐ 2. Clinician reports that patient B needs Social Service intervention.

☐ 3. Clinician determines whether patient can demonstrate the proper use of oxygen equipment by visit three.

☐ 4. Clinician performs a respiratory assessment.

☐ 5. Clinician and patient decide on the following goal:
Patient will describe five acceptable ways to minimize anxiety prior to discharge.

*Answers: 1, 3, and 5.*
*Rationale: Outcome indicators are written in objective terms, yielding a quantified measurement in percentages, averages, means, or scores.*

---

## When and by Whom are Outcome Measurements Made?

To be most effective, outcome measurements should by integrated into routine care processes (Kleinpell, 2003) and measured by clinicians who provide care (Hill, 1999). Mandates for measuring OASIS outcomes specify that certain skilled disciplines complete assessment items at specific points in time (CMS, 2002b).

Not all OASIS items are collected or measured at every time point. For example, because the OASIS Adverse Event outcome, *Emergent care for hypo/hyperglycemia*, is documented to reflect the need for emergent care after the patient has been admitted to home care, it is not included in the OASIS admission data set items.

When an agency measures outcomes in addition to OASIS, the agency decides who should measure these outcomes and when the outcomes are to be measured. For example, a physical therapist is likely to be more qualified to measure an outcome that requires the use of a *functional measurement* scale. An LPN/LVN is equally as qualified as the RN to measure the patient's verbalization of the importance of compliance with fluid restriction.

Following are examples of timeframes used for end measurements of agency-written educational, compliance, and clinical outcomes. Each discusses the rationale for the selection.

### Example 1

Patient/caretaker will verbalize risk factors for heart disease **by discharge.**

This timeframe indicates that the clinician can measure or determine if the patient can verbalize this information anytime up to and including discharge.

*Rationale: The subject matter is not urgently required of the patient or caretaker and can be taught later in the episode of care.*

### Example 2

The patient/caretaker verbalizes adverse signs and symptoms to report **by visit three.**

The outcome is measured by the clinician no later than visit three.

*Rationale: The subject matter can potentially help the patient avoid harmful consequences and is taught earlier in the episode.*

### Example 3

Patient is compliant with the home exercise program *while on service.*

This timeframe indicates that the outcome is measured periodically while patient is receiving homecare services, culminating in a single measurement for the patient when service is ended; or a single measurement is made at the time when service is ended.

*Rationale: Compliance with the subject matter is not evaluated until the subject matter is taught. Compliance is measured from this point forward.*

## Documenting Outcome Measurements

Outcome measurements are typically documented through the use of data gathering tools, such as flowcharts, check sheets, pathways, and data collection forms, or through the use of valid and reliable instruments (Kleinpell, 2003), as in the case of OASIS.

### Example 1

For OASIS outcomes, the clinician documents patient responses to OASIS items, making observations or entering descriptions using OASIS data set item response instructions as the guide. For example, OASIS item *(M0420) Frequency of Pain* is documented by the clinician on admission as #3 = all of the time. At discharge, the assessment of the item is #1 = less often than daily. These documented responses are keyed into OASIS software, where the outcome is calculated for the patient and presented in an OBQI outcome report.

### Example 2

The clinician documents the measurement of an individual patient outcome indicator as *Met, Not Met,* or *Not Applicable.* This method is commonly used in care pathway design. For example, your agency developed the following outcome indicator: *Patient/caretaker verbalizes the safe and proper use of oxygen equipment within two weeks.*

An assessment of patient/caretaker knowledge is made on or soon after admission. Patient teaching is then carried out. If the patient can verbalize safe and proper use of oxygen equipment within two weeks, the clinician documents the outcome as *Met.* If the patient cannot verbalize this information within two weeks, the outcome is documented as *Not Met.* If this outcome is part of the agency COPD pathway and the patient is not using oxygen, the outcome will be measured as *Not Applicable.* An evaluation of each outcome is made and documented based on its specified timeframe.

### Example 3

The Likert scale, used in the Outcomes Classification Project (Moorehead, Johnson, and Maas, 2004), requires that the clinician circle the number most representative of the individual's ability, actions, or understanding of the outcome indicator in question. The documentation of responses culminates in an outcome for each indicator measured.

*Example 4*

Another method documents outcomes as diagnostic values, degrees of movement, adverse events, or physiological findings, such as finger-stick blood sugars or blood pressure. For example, a functional measurement scale is used to document flexion and extension in patients with total knee replacement, at admission and discharge. The degree of change is documented as the outcome for the patient.

1A

## Accuracy of Outcome Measurements

Accuracy in measuring outcomes is critical for obtaining meaningful and usable outcomes data. Data are the foundation of analyses, all of which are flawed if the data are filled with inaccuracies (Jennings and Staggers, 1999). While this is particularly obvious for outcomes data for quality of care, financial and marketing outcomes are also affected.

Accurate data should be an obvious concern for everyone involved in outcome measurement (Kraus and Horan, 1997). Zuber (2002) raises concerns about inaccurate OASIS data collection and strongly suggests that managers and clinicians give proper attention to it. The clinician must use the OASIS response instructions provided by CMS to describe a patient's health status accurately.

For example, a clinician assesses a patient's health status for OASIS item *(M0490): When is the patient dyspneic or noticeably short of breath?* while the patient is on oxygen. The patient uses oxygen intermittently. The OASIS instructions state that if a patient uses oxygen intermittently, the clinician is to mark the item that best describes the patient's shortness of breath *without* the use of oxygen (CMS, 2002b). In this case, the response given by the clinician is not an *accurate* one and yields flawed data.

In this same example, not only will the outcomes for quality of care be flawed, but the financial data are flawed as well. Let's examine how. The patient uses oxygen intermittently. However, if the clinician assesses *M0490: When is the patient noticeably short of breath?* with the patient's oxygen on and the patient is assessed as #1 (Dyspneic or Short of Breath when walking 20 feet, climbing stairs), reimbursement will be less than what it actually should be.

Imagine this one flaw multiplied by many. Not only are the financial outcomes data flawed for future comparisons, but the reimbursement needed to manage patient care is also less than is needed. If inaccurate OASIS outcome measurements are substantial, the agency's financial status can be severely impacted.

On a larger scale, the aggregate of inaccurate responses has the potential to make an agency's outcomes data appear better or worse than they actually are. Both result in incorrect conclusions and inaccurate comparisons of the agency's data to other agencies. In addition, both can affect reference group data. If agencies in a reference group document an OASIS response incorrectly, reference data are not accurate and comparisons are rendered meaningless.

Agency management can ensure the accuracy of outcome measurements and resulting outcomes data in several ways. Clinician education, clinical record audits, data entry audits, and home visit observation are helpful methods to establish or verify accuracy of OASIS outcomes (CMS, 2002b) and financial outcomes data. While these methods are recommended for OASIS responses, they can also serve as excellent guidelines for agency supplemental outcome measurements. Incorporate them into care processes and performance improvement initiatives on a regular basis.

*Clinician education* helps to outline staff expectations regarding their role in outcomes measurement. Include illustrations of various OASIS items and their corresponding definitions, as well as the effect of inaccurate responses on outcomes data published in agency outcome reports. Address potential financial implications. Review agency definitions and procedure for care pathway outcome measurements, if applicable.

*Clinical record audits* enable you to compare outcome measurements to interventions provided and to determine if discrepancies exist within the documentation. Patient responses may be inaccurately evaluated, resulting in an incorrect Request for Anticipated Payment (RAP).

For example, the patient response to *M0420: Frequency of Pain* is #3—all of the time, yet there is no pain medication or other interventions mentioned to relieve pain. The patient's M0245 diagnosis is hypertension. This appears to be a discrepancy. If the evaluation of the patient's response is incorrect, then the RAP can be wrong. Both clinical and financial outcomes are affected for this patient.

The patient response to *M0490: When is the patient short of breath?* documented by the nurse is #1—when walking more than 20 feet, yet the physical therapist documents in her evaluation that dyspnea does not occur until the patient walks 100 feet. Both the clinical and financial outcomes are affected.

*Data entry audits* reveal an error that occurs between the responses recorded by staff and the responses that are recorded by data entry. Errors are checked by conducting an audit of a small sample of records at monthly intervals (CMS, 2002b). The errors can be converted to a percent and tracked over time to stay abreast of the error rate. This method is especially helpful when new processes are implemented or when new employees begin data entry.

*Home visit observation* allows senior and managerial staff to conduct periodic home visits with clinicians to evaluate whether appropriate definitions for outcome measurements are used. These home visits allow staff with expertise in outcome measurement to provide on-site assistance at the time of data collection.

### Guiding Questions

For OASIS outcome measurements:
- Are staff using correct response instructions of OASIS items to elicit responses?
- Is the right discipline assessing the right data set items at the right time?
- Does clinical visit note documentation correspond with OASIS responses?

For agency supplemental outcome measurements:
- Are staff measuring the outcomes according to agency definition?
- Do interventions coincide with agency standards of care?

## ESTABLISHING RELIABILITY AND VALIDITY OF OUTCOME INDICATORS (MEASURES)

The quality of outcomes data is not only affected by accuracy of measurement, but also by the design of the outcome measures themselves. If your agency writes some of its own outcome indicators, you should determine the validity and reliability of these measures prior to clinical use.

### Validity

Merriam-Webster (2002) defines *valid* as that which is meaningful, appropriate to the end, well grounded, or true. Outcomes data must be meaningful and true for use and application. For example, the measurement of the complication rate of central line insertions in an intensive care unit is a *valid* or *meaningful* outcome indicator for a hospital, but is *not valid* or *meaningful* for a homecare agency.

Outcomes must also be measured accurately to be valid. Polit, Beck, and Hungler (2001) and Linacre (2000) state that data are considered valid if they actually measure what they are supposed to measure. If the measurements are not valid, the outcomes attained have no real meaning, and the outcomes data will be inappropriately skewed and/or applied. While there are a number of approaches to assessing the validity of outcome indicators (measures), we will focus on three criteria that are frequently used: content validity, construct validity, and criterion-related validity.

*Content validity* can be determined by asking the question, *"Do the outcome indicators adequately cover the subject matter being measured?"* This question is particularly relevant for measures of knowledge and psychosocial traits (Polit, Beck, and Hungler, 2001). This question is subjective and is generally assessed by experts in the subject or by literature review. For example, the *content validity* of outcome indicators related to the care provided to newly diagnosed diabetic patients would be questioned if these indicators did not include recognition of signs and symptoms of hypo/hyperglycemia.

*Construct validity* is more difficult to establish. One approach compares groups that are expected to differ in a critical attribute or outcome measure. Let's assess the construct validity of the outcome indicator, *Patient/caretaker verbalizes the signs and symptoms of hypo/hyperglycemia and how to treat.* Clinicians measure this outcome indicator in a group of newly diagnosed diabetic patients two days after instruction is completed. They also measure this same indicator in a group of patients who have had diabetes for 10 years or more. We expect the patients who are newly diagnosed to score lower. If this difference is not exhibited, the construct validity of this outcome is questioned.

*Criterion-related validity* is the degree to which *responses of different patients to the outcome indicator correlate with external criteria* (Polit, Beck, and Hungler, 2001). For example, do the responses of newly diagnosed diabetic patients for the outcome indicator, *verbalizes signs and symptoms of hypo/hyperglycemia,* correlate with the external criteria of *verbalizes special dietary considerations?* In other words, a patient with newly diagnosed diabetes would be expected to score similarly on both of these indicators.

## Reliability

Reliability refers to *the consistency and accuracy of a measure* (Polit, Beck, and Hungler, 2001; Linacre, 2000). A measure is considered reliable if it is consistently reproducible. The less variation an instrument produces in repeated measurements of an attribute or outcome indicator, the higher its reliability (Polit, Beck, and Hungler, 2001). For example, a patient steps on a scale and weighs 140 pounds. He weighs again in ten minutes and the scale displays a reading of 156 pounds. He weighs again in five minutes and the scale displays 148 pounds. This measure is considered *unreliable.*

Let's look at an example that demonstrates the importance of using a *reliable* outcomes measurement tool. The following outcome is an excerpt from an outcomes measurement tool for the patient with a fracture:

*Patient/caretaker verbalizes the elements of a neurological/circulatory assessment by the second visit.*

One measures the outcome as *Met* if the patient verbalizes the elements of blanching and sensation. This clinician bases the patient's outcome measurement on these two elements only. Another clinician measures the outcome as *Not Met* if the patient verbalizes *only* the elements of blanching and sensation. This clinician bases the outcome measurement on five elements of the assessment. Different clinicians measure the patient's outcomes differently.

Notice that the tool does not specify what the neurological/circulatory assessment should consist of, and no other instructions exist to guide the clinician's measurement of this indicator. This allows different clinicians to use their own *definitions* of neurological/circulatory assessment in measuring this outcome. This results in two diametrically opposed outcome measurements, originating from an unreliable outcome indicator. How can we make this outcome indicator or measure reliable? The reliability of the indicator is enhanced if:

1. the outcome indicator specifies the items to be assessed,
2. items are included as part of patient teaching material for reference by the clinician, or if
3. items are included in a definition format for easy access by the clinician.

However, the only way to know for sure is to conduct reliability testing of the indicator.

Reliability is determined statistically by a number of different methods, referred to as reliability testing. Two of these are *inter-rater reliability* and *intra-rater reliability*.

***Inter-rater reliability*** is obtained by having two raters use the same instrument to independently collect data at the same time (Polit, Beck, and Hungler, 2001). For example, two clinicians observe and independently document patient responses for the Start of Care OASIS data set items during the same home visit. Inter-rater reliability determines the extent to which the documentation of both clinicians is in agreement.

***Intra-rater reliability*** is obtained by having one rater complete the same instrument at different times. For example, the same clinician completes the same OASIS data set items at two different times. Intra-rater reliability determines the extent to which the responses are the same, given the same set of circumstances at two different times.

## Using Reliable Tools

The OASIS data set items are considered *reliable* measurements of OASIS data, as substantial reliability has been demonstrated (Madigan, 2002). OASIS items have specific parameters outlined within that guide clinicians in their documentation of each item. Handbooks are also available that provide more in-depth OASIS response instructions for use (CMS, 2002a).

There are a growing number of other measurement tools that have been formally tested and deemed reliable for collecting agency supplemental outcomes data. These include:

- the Wong-Baker Faces scale that measures pain intensity (Polit, Beck, and Hungler, 2001)
- the State Trait Anxiety Inventory that measures anxiety
- the Arthritis Impact Measurement Scale (AIMS) that measures the impact of arthritis
- the Functional Independence Measure (FIM)
- the Medical Outcomes Study Short Form 36 (SF-36) (Arslanian, 2001)
- the Nursing Outcomes Classification (NOC) (Moorehead, Johnson, and Mass, 2004)

It is recommended that you use tested, reliable measurement tools whenever possible (Whittington, 1998). However, if you design your own measurement tools to capture agency supplemental outcomes data in addition to OASIS outcomes, you must give attention to the reliability of the indicators or measures that you write.

*Testing* the reliability of any instrument includes the application of sophisticated statistical methods. It is advised that you seek the assistance and expertise of one who has knowledge in this area, as presentation of these methods is beyond the scope of this text. A college campus is an excellent place to begin your search for a professor, instructor, or graduate student assistant who teaches statistics or research methodology. They have the ability you seek. Also, masters prepared nurses usually have the statistics background to conduct simple reliability testing.

**1A**

## CONCEPT APPLICATION:
### Enhancing the Reliability of Outcome Indicators

Examine the following outcome measure:

*Patient/caretaker verbalizes the elements of a neurological/circulatory assessment by the second visit.*

Identify the following items that improve the reliability of this outcome indicator:

☐ 1. Conduct a follow-up class on neurological/circulatory assessment of a fractured extremity.

☐ 2. Include the elements of the neurological/circulatory assessment within the outcome measurement tool.

☐ 3. Require the use of standardized patient teaching sheets for use with all patients with fractures. These sheets include the five components of an acceptable neurological/circulatory assessment.

☐ 4. Conduct reliability testing of the tool.

*Answer: 2, 3, and 4.*
*Rationale: While educational classes are helpful, a clinician must rely on memory alone to know exactly what is to be assessed.*

## OUTCOME REPORTS

An outcome report reflects results of outcomes measured over a particular period of time and aggregated (totaled) to the agency level (CMS, 2002b). It displays percentages of patients who have achieved and not achieved the measured outcomes. The agency uses an outcome report to select or *target* particular outcomes for performance improvement.

For the purpose of comparison, the OASIS OBQI outcome reports include outcomes data from a national reference group and from the agency's prior time period. State OASIS software applications automatically generate OASIS OBQI outcome reports. OASIS outcome reports are also available through privatized data warehouses.

An agency can design and generate its own outcome reports for those outcomes that it writes or for outcomes that are measured through purchased care pathways. These reports can be produced manually or through agency software applications, and designed to aggregate percentages of outcomes achieved, not achieved, or not applicable according to pre-defined patient specifics. These include demographics, diagnosis or condition, location of residence, primary language, co-morbid condition(s), referral source, and others.

# INTERNAL AND EXTERNAL BENCHMARKING OF OUTCOMES DATA

Benchmarking is *the use of a point of reference by which others are judged* (Merriam-Webster, 2002). Wilson and Nathan (2003) describe it as a sighting point from which a measurement is made or a standard against which others are measured. The Benchmarking Exchange (2003) defines it as the process of identifying, understanding, and adapting outstanding practices from organizations to help your own organization improve its performance.

Benchmarking entails collecting and comparing performance data and information to identify the operational and clinical practices that lead to best outcomes (Rosswurm and Larrabee, 1999).

These data can include clinical findings, physician practice profiles, state, regional, and national standards and averages, managed care contract data, resource utilization, financial indicators, and staffing and productivity (Strassner, 1997). Walker, Houston, and LeClair (1997) state that benchmarking is essential to maintain a broader perspective on healthcare services provided. Benchmarking allows an entity to make data comparisons within the organization *(internal benchmarking)*, and to compare itself to other organizations using like indicators *(external benchmarking)*.

As prospective payment systems have compelled agencies to improve efficiency in care delivery (Lagoe, Noetscher, and Murphy, 2000), benchmarking has become a necessity for healthcare organizations to maintain and achieve desired levels of quality. One of the best ways to benchmark an organization's quality is through the benchmarking of outcomes data (Wilson and Nathan, 2003).

## Internal Benchmarking

Comparing one's current data to a prior period is as important as comparing current data to outside entities. There are several ways to perform internal benchmarking. An agency's OASIS outcomes data can now be compared to prior periods through OBQI reports that reflect the agency's data past and present. Comparative data are also made available to agencies through companies that specialize in warehousing outcomes data. Member agencies can generate comparative reports for use. Agencies can also benchmark local data generated in one department to similar data generated in another.

Large homecare companies with multiple providers, who measure identical outcomes, can use internal benchmarking to compare results among sister agencies. Internal benchmarking is especially easy in this case because business and performance improvement strategies can be shared without fear of compromising market position.

Examples of internal benchmarking include:

- A corporate homecare company that systematically compares its sister agencies' financial and clinical outcomes data, including satisfaction, OASIS outcomes data, and agency marketing data.
- An individual agency that compares its monthly supply use and costs for the patient with stasis ulcers to an acceptable in-house company goal.

## External Benchmarking

For some time now, homecare providers have benchmarked agency information against data provided by national, state, and independent associations. As outcomes data have moved to the forefront in quality improvement, companies that warehouse outcomes data for member use are on the rise. These companies provide valuable outcomes data in a myriad of ways, including those specified by the individual member agency.

Some companies send periodic surveys to agency members to ascertain financial, productivity, and staffing mix data. These data are aggregated and provided to agency members for external benchmarking purposes. Practitioners examine internal data and assess the need for a change in practice by comparing these data with external data provided by these benchmarking databases (Rosswurm and Larabee, 1999).

Examples of external benchmarking include:

- An agency that compares its own average of SN visits per episode for the patient with CHF to a national average of 14.
- A company that warehouses outcomes data provides financial information that includes annual salary information of executives and staff clinicians for each region of the country. An agency provider-member compares its information to its own region's benchmarks.
- An agency's review of its OBQI Adverse Event Outcome Report shows that 2.8% of its patients had the outcome of *Development of urinary tract infection* as compared to the national reference (all Medicare-certified homecare agencies) of 1.2% for the same outcome. The agency evaluates its results of 2.8% against the national reference (the external benchmark) of 1.2%.

1A

---

### CONCEPT APPLICATION:
### Identifying Internal and External Benchmarks

Identify the following benchmarks as internal or external:

**INT. EXT.**

☐ ☐  1. National rate of CHF hospital re-admissions

☐ ☐  2. Comparison of agency satisfaction data to corporate average

☐ ☐  3. Regional salary range of nurse middle managers

☐ ☐  4. Average national reimbursement for a particular HHRG

☐ ☐  5. Comparison of data entry audit errors against the company's acceptable threshold

*Answers: 1. External  2. Internal  3. External  4. External  5. Internal*
*Rationale: Data comparison to benchmarks outside a homecare company or an independent agency is external benchmarking. Data comparison within is internal.*

## AGENCY APPLICATION:
### Identifying Agency Benchmarks

Identify five **internal** benchmarks that your agency can use for comparison.

1._____

2._____

3._____

4._____

5._____

Identify five **external** benchmarks available for use that are pertinent to your agency's patient populations.

1._____

2._____

3._____

4._____

5._____

## REFERENCES

Arslanian, C. (2001). Developing an orthopaedic outcomes program. *Orthopaedic Nursing*, 20(2), 19. Retrieved April 16, 2003 from Infotrac database.

Blancett, S. & Flarey, D. (1998). *Health care outcomes: Collaborative, path-based approaches.* Gaithersburg, MD: Aspen.

Camann, M. A. (2001). Outcomes of care: The use of conceptual models to "see the forest and the trees" in planning outcomes studies. *Topics in Health Information Management*, 22(2), 10. Retrieved June 27, 2003 from Infotrac database.

Centers for Medicare and Medicaid Services, U.S. Department of Health and Human Services. (2002a). Oasis in detail: A clinician's pocket guide. Briggs Corporation.

Centers for Medicare and Medicaid Services, U.S. Department of Health and Human Services. (2002b). Outcome-based quality improvement (OBQI) implementation manual. Baltimore, MD: author.

Cleemput, I. & Kestlefoot, K. (2002). Economic implications of non-compliance in health care. *The Lancet*, 359(9324), 2129. Retrieved January 8, 2003 from Infotrac database.

Cramer, J. A. (2002). Effect of partial compliance on cardiovascular medication effectiveness. *Heart*, 88(2), 203. Retrieved June 27, 2003 from Infotrac database.

Crisler, K.S., Baillie, L., & Conway, K. (2003). Using new OASIS-based reports in OBQI. *Home Healthcare Nurse*, 21(9), 621–626.

Critical pathways: An acute care tool enters the homecare setting. (1994). *Hospital Home Care*, 11(1), 1–12.

Epstein, R. S. & Sherwood, L. M. (1996). From outcomes research to disease management: A guide for the perplexed. *Annals of Internal Medicine*, 124(9), 832. Retrieved April 16, 2003 from Infotrac database.

Hill, M. (1999). Outcomes measurement requires nursing to shift to outcome-based practice. *Nursing Administration Quarterly*, 24(1), 1. Retrieved January 14, 2003 from Infotrac database.

Humphrey, C. J. & Malone-Nuzzo, P. (1996). *Orientation to home care nursing.* Gaithersburg, MD: Aspen.

Jennings, B. M., Staggers, N., & Brosch, L. R. (1999). A classification scheme for outcome indicators. *Journal of Nursing Scholarship*, 31(4), 381. Retrieved January 10, 2003 from Infotrac database.

Johlin, F. C. (1999). Perspective from a physician. University of Iowa Hospitals and Clinics: Outcomes management. *Nursing Administration Quarterly*, 24(1), 31. Retrieved April 16, 2003 from Infotrac database.

Kleinpell, R. M. (2003). Measuring advanced practice nursing outcomes: Strategies and resources. *Critical Care Nurse*, 23(1), S6.

Kraus, D. R. & Horan, F. P. (1997). Outcomes roadblocks: Problems and solutions. *Behavioral Health Management*, 17(5), 22. Retrieved June 27, 2003 from Infotrac database.

Lagoe, R. L., Noetscher, C. M., & Murphy, M. E. (2000). Combined benchmarking of hospital outcomes and utilization. *Nursing Economics*, 18(2), NA.

Lamb-Harvard, J. (1997). Nurses at the bedside: Influencing outcomes. In S. Prevost (Ed.), *The Nursing Clinics of North America: Outcomes and outcome measurement* (pp. 579–587). Philadelphia: W. B. Saunders.

Linacre, J. M. (2000). New approaches to determining reliability and validity. *Research Quarterly for Exercise and Sport*, 71(2), 129. Retrieved April 14, 2003 from Infotrac database.

Madigan, E. A. (2002). The scientific dimensions of OASIS for home care outcome measurement. *Home Healthcare Nurse*, 20(9), 579–583.

Mensing, C., Boucher, J., Cypress, M., Weigner, K., Mulcahy, K., Barta, P. et al. (2003). National standards for diabetes self-management education. *Diabetes Care*, 26, (S149–S156). Retrieved August 8, 2003 from http://care.diabetesjournals.|org/cgi/content/full/26/suppl_1/S149#SEC7.

Merboth, M. K. & Barnason, S. (2000). Managing pain: The fifth vital sign. *The Nursing Clinics of North America. Chronic disease self-management: Improving health outcomes*, 35(2), 375–383.

*Merriam-Webster's Collegiate Dictionary (10th ed.).* (2002). Merriam-Webster, Inc.

Moorehead, S., Johnson, M., & Maas, M. (Eds.). (2004). *Nursing outcomes classification (NOC).* St. Louis, MO: Mosby.

Outcomes Research. (March 2000). [Fact Sheet]. AHRQ Publication No. 00-P011. Agency for Healthcare Research and Quality, Rockville, MD. http://www.hrq.gov/clinic/outfact.htm.

Peters, C., Cowley, M., & Standiford, L. (1999). The process of outcomes management in an acute care facility. *Nursing Administration Quarterly*, 24(1), 75. Retrieved January 8, 2003 from Infotrac database.

Polit, D., Beck, C.T., & Hungler, B. P. (2001). *Essentials of nursing research: Methods, appraisal, and utilization.* Philadelphia: Lippincott, Williams and Wilkins.

Renders, C. M., Gerlof, D.V., Simon, J. G., Wagner, E. H., Ejik Van, J. T., & Assendelft, W. J. (2001). Interventions to improve the management of diabetes in primary care, outpatient, and community settings. *Diabetes Care*, 24(10), 1821. Retrieved January 8, 2003 from Infotrac database.

Rosswurm, M. A. & Larrabee, J. H. (1999). A model for change to evidence-based practice. *Image: Journal of Nursing Scholarship*, 31(4), 317. Retrieved January 8, 2003 from Infotrac database.

Shaughnessy, P. W., Crisler, K. S., & Schlenker, R. (1997). Medicare's OASIS: Standardized outcome and assessment information set for Home Care care. Denver, Colorado: The University of Colorado, Center for Health Services and Policy Research.

Sidorov, J. (2003). Building your own DM initiative. Disease Management Association of America [featured lecture]. Retrieved June 14, 2003 from http://www.dmaa.org/2003conference/sidorov.pdf.

Strassner, L. (1997). Critical pathways: The next generation of outcomes tracking. *Orthopaedic Nursing*, 16(2), S56.

Strickland, O. L. (1997). Challenges in measuring patient outcomes. In S. Prevost (Ed.), *The Nursing Clinics of North America: Outcomes and outcome measurement* (pp. 495–512). Philadelphia: W. B. Saunders.

The Benchmarking Exchange. (2003). What is benchmarking? Retrieved December 6, 2003 from http://www.benchmarking.org/wib.

Waggoner, M. G. (1999). Clinical pathways: From the hospital to the home. *Med-Surg Nursing*, 8(4), 265. Retrieved May 16, 2003 from Infotrac database.

Walker, D., Houston, S., & LeClair, C. (1997). Outcomes management in orthopedics. In S. Prevost (Ed.), *The Nursing Clinics of North America: Outcomes and outcome management* (pp. 561–569). Philadelphia: W. B. Saunders.

Whittington, C. F. (1998). Outcomes management: Who, what, where, why, how. *Orthopaedic Nursing*, 17(2), S15.

Wilson, A. & Nathan, L. (2003). Understanding benchmarks. *Home Healthcare Nurse*, 21(2), 102–107.

Zuber, R. F. (2002). Oasis data quality needs attention. *Home Healthcare Nurse*, 20(11), 756.

**1**A

# The Foundation of Outcome-Based Home Care: Outcomes Measurement and Standards of Care

Section B

## Variance and Variance Management

### CORE TERMS AND CONCEPTS

- Variance
- Variance Management
- Variance Data
- Positive Variance
- Negative Variance
- Aggregation of Variance Data
- Variance Analysis

### LEARNING OBJECTIVES

Upon completion of this topic, you will able to:

1. Define variance.
2. Identify causes of variance.
3. Describe activities in variance management.
4. Aggregate and trend variance data.
5. Perform variance analysis.

### AGENCY-SPECIFIC DATA/RESOURCES NEEDED

Agency variance data currently in use, if applicable

# INTRODUCTION

Addressing variance in patient treatment, recovery, and response is not new to home care clinicians. We are accustomed to assisting the patient and caretaker(s) when unexpected delays in treatment and recovery occur, or when the patient's response *varies* from the norm. We address and resolve each patient's situation as much as possible, primarily on an individual basis. However, as we move to an outcome-based approach to home care, we have an additional question to ask about variations in patient responses: How do these variations affect outcomes achieved?

# WHAT IS VARIANCE?

In health care, *variance* is most often seen as a component of care pathways, thus affecting the patient's ability to attain desired outcomes (Fuss and Pasquale, 1998; Porrier and Oberleitner, 1999) within the timeframe for which a care pathway is designed (Strassner, 1997). Variance can also be documented as a deviation from the number of planned visits according to the plan of care or as a deviation from the patient's anticipated response to treatment.

Variance is defined by Agnes (2003) as *a state or quality varying or changing from the standard*. Variance can be positive or negative, even though most healthcare variances tracked are negative. A patient has varied *positively* from a pathway or planned intervention when he or she is discharged with *outcomes met earlier* than the number of visits planned. A patient has varied *negatively* from the pathway or planned interventions when *outcomes are not met as anticipated* in the number of visits planned.

# CAUSES OF VARIANCE

Reasons that patients vary negatively from planned interventions or visits may include, but are not limited to:

- Multiple caretakers
- Difficulty in reading/writing English
- Financial barriers to treatment
- Poor hygienic environment
- Two or more newly prescribed medications
- Medical complication
- Lack of caretaker/family support
- New infection since admission
- Noncompliance
- Fall with injury

Reasons that patients vary positively from planned interventions or visits may include, but are not limited to:

- No medical complications
- Considerable caretaker/family support
- Two or less consistent caretakers
- Previously acquired knowledge of self-management skills

Let's look at some examples of outcomes to see how these may be affected by variance. OASIS outcomes *Improvement in Ambulation* and *Improvement in Transfer* may be adversely affected if the patient suffers a fall with injury while on service. This occurrence may result in patient decline or in an extended length of stay and may prevent the outcomes from being achieved in the original timeframe. If this occurs, the fall with injury is considered a reason for patient variance.

An agency written outcome, *Patient/caretaker demonstrates proper wound management within four weeks,* can be adversely affected if multiple caretakers are providing care. Multiple caretakers may require more home visits for teaching, spanning eight weeks, as opposed to the four weeks originally planned.

---

### CONCEPT APPLICATION:
### Identifying Reasons for Variance

Select the three reasons for variance from the following list:

☐ Blindness

☐ Patient assessment

☐ Language barrier

☐ Staff dog bite

☐ Lack of money for medicine/treatment

*Answers: Blindness, Language barrier, and Lack of money for medicine/treatment. Rationale: These reasons for variance can affect a patient's length of stay and outcomes achieved.*

Identify two additional causes of variance that have not been mentioned in this discussion.

1. _____

2. _____

---

## REPORTING/DOCUMENTING CAUSES OF VARIANCE

Variance in the patient care setting must either be verbally reported or documented by staff. Staff should report or document variance (cause of variance) on the visit or day it is noted so this information does not go unreported.

Evaluate your current processes of daily clinical information flow regarding patient care. Also look at the documentation that your agency requires of staff on a daily basis. Variance can be *reported* via verbal exchange with specific office personnel. (Include variance in the staff's *daily report* to supervisory personnel.)

Variance can be *documented* via:

• Written communication note. (Use a *special note* or notation designed for communicating variance.)
• Documentation within clinical forms/software. (Dedicate a special area within clinical forms/software for the documentation of variance.)

Regardless of the method that your agency employs to report variance, staying abreast of staff compliance with the process and reiterating its importance will be a key to having the variance data needed to give perspective to outcomes achieved.

*Guiding Questions*

- What are causes of variance that are likely to affect the ability of our patients to achieve the outcomes we desire?
- Can variance be added to the current method of reporting?
- Can variance be documented on current forms that are processed through data entry on a daily basis? Can data entry input the variance data at this time?
- What are the reasons for variance that are most applicable to the patients that we care for?

---

### AGENCY APPLICATION:
### Reporting and Documenting Variance

How will the agency capture variance? _____

_____

Reporting: When and how often? _____

_____

Documenting: When and how often? _____

_____

---

## VARIANCE MANAGEMENT

Variance management is *the identification of causes of variance and the action taken to minimize or eliminate its effect on patient progress.* Variance management is two-fold. It occurs both at the patient level and at the agency level (Hill, 1999). At the patient level, causes of variance are identified and addressed concurrently while patient is on service. The clinician identifying the cause can address it with the patient and caretaker(s), discuss options with the manager or director, or discuss the patient during case conference as appropriate. This type of variance management is conducted in some form almost daily.

At the agency level, variance is aggregated for all patients over a period of time and is retrospectively studied and evaluated to determine overall effects on selected patient groups or diagnoses. It involves identifying, collecting, reporting, and analyzing variance and its related causes (Hill, 1999). These activities are designed to discover opportunities for PI where modifications are made in care delivery, care pathway components, and/or planning of visits.

## AGGREGATION OF VARIANCE DATA

We are accustomed to recognizing and addressing reasons why a patient does not progress on an individual basis. Additionally, we have learned that variance management is employed at the agency level to evaluate these reasons and their effect on overall outcomes achieved by the agency. However, while reasons for variance should be documented and addressed for the individual patient, not all causes of variance are aggregated or monitored for their effects on overall agency outcomes (Hill, 1999). This is to prevent a plethora of unnecessary data collection.

Aggregation of variance data is one method of variance management. Aggregation is a group of distinct things gathered into a total (Agnes, 2003). Aggregation of variance data expresses a total percentage for each cause of variance occurring in a specific patient population over a specific period of time. Aggregation of variance data gives perspective to outcome percentages and helps to pinpoint areas of possible cause on a larger scale.

For example, an agency has an increase in surgical wound infections. Fifty-two percent of the patients with surgical wound infections require an average of 16 additional visits. Aggregation of the variance data reveals that 58% of all patients admitted with a diagnosis of surgical wound *live in a poor hygienic environment*, and 46% are *non-compliant* with frequency of dressing changes.

In a second example, an agency has less than desirable outcomes for compliance with insulin management. Aggregation of variance data shows that 38% of all patients admitted with a diagnosis of diabetes in the last year had *financial barriers to treatment*. Thirty-four percent of these patients required an average of eight additional visits resulting from financial constraints.

How does an agency select variances for aggregation?

- Consider your agency's high volume, high risk, or problematic diagnoses as you select variance data for overall aggregation.
- Review current quality indicators that are used in performance improvement, and determine which ones are value-added versus non-value added (Strassner, 1997).
- Consider the outcomes that you deem important for your patients to achieve, and determine if the variances you are considering will help in the analysis of these particular outcomes.

## Manual Aggregation of Variance Data

Aggregation may be accomplished manually or through automation. Automation is by far the more efficient of the two. You and your computer programmer need to understand the manual calculations to effectively collaborate on developing your software application correctly.

Aggregate each reason for variance for a particular time period. Quarterly aggregation is recommended; larger agencies may find monthly aggregation more manageable. Annual aggregation of variance data is also recommended.

## CONCEPT APPLICATION:
### Aggregating Causes of Variance

The following is an excerpt of variances that Agency A has chosen to document and aggregate:

- Patient fall with injury

- New infection post admission

- Financial barriers to treatment

For the month of April/year XXXX
Total patients discharged in April: 50

| Reasons for Variance | Total # | Total # of Variances of One Type Divided by # of Patients | % Variance Reported |
|---|---|---|---|
| Patient fall with injury: | 6 | 6/50 = | 12% |
| New infection post admission: | 4 | 4/50 = | 8% |
| Financial barriers to treatment: | 8 | 8/50 = | 16% |

## AGENCY APPLICATION:
### Selecting a Method of Aggregation

Will your agency aggregate variance manually or through automation?

_____

_____

## TRENDING OF VARIANCE DATA

Variance data are trended through the same process as that for outcomes data. The aggregated variance percentages are reported for each month or quarter respectively. Findings are compared and contrasted month-to-month or quarter-to-quarter.

## USE OF VARIANCE IN ANALYZING PATIENT OUTCOMES DATA

Variance helps to analyze outcomes achieved by giving perspective to your investigation and by providing areas of concern for further investigation and revision. Variance aggregation is reviewed along with the outcome results for the same period. They go hand-in-hand. For example, an agency's OASIS Adverse Event outcome of *Emergent care for wound infections, deteriorating wound status* is significantly higher than the national reference sample for the first six months of the year. The agency's variance data for *multiple caretakers* is 38% for patients with pressure ulcers during this same time period. Upon further investigation and chart review, the agency finds that the majority of patients experiencing this adverse event outcome also had a poor hygienic environment.

The agency concludes that these two factors played a major role in the deterioration of these patients' wounds. The agency further discusses ways to enhance wound care provided in this type of situation and to consider alternative care provision as appropriate.

---

### CONCEPT APPLICATION:
#### Use of Variance to Analyze Outcomes Data

An agency **measures the outcome**: patient demonstrates proper use of diary to record food intake while on service. Only 69% of patients with diagnoses related to malabsorption conditions achieved this outcome in the last six months. Therefore, the outcome is not being met adequately based on agency expectations.

The investigation reveals that the low percentage has occurred primarily in a geographical area where literacy is a problem. For this same patient population, the variance data for *difficulty in reading/writing English* are reported at 82%. This leads the agency to target patient/caretaker education as a possible contributor to this problem.

The agency brainstorms with staff and decides to review and possibly revise educational methods and materials used to teach patients/caretakers with reading and/or writing difficulty. When the agency makes these revisions in the patient education methods, a follow-up evaluation is made to see if the outcome for patients in this geographical area has improved.

---

1B

---

## AGENCY APPLICATION:
### Selecting Causes of Variance

List causes of variance that your agency will consider for aggregation.

_____

_____

_____

_____

_____

_____

---

### REFERENCES

Agnes, M. (Ed.). (2003). *Webster's New World College Dictionary (4th ed.)*. NY: Macmillan.

Fuss, M. A. & Pasquale, M. D. (1998). Clinical management protocols: The bedside answer to clinical practice guidelines. *Journal of Trauma Nursing*, 5(1), 10. Retrieved June 27, 2003 from Infotrac database.

Hill, M. (1999). Outcomes measurement requires nursing to shift to outcome-based practice. *Nursing Administration Quarterly*, 24(1), 1–9. Retrieved January 8, 2003 from Infotrac database.

Porrier, G. & Oberleitner, M. G. (1999). *Clinical pathways in nursing: A guide to managing care from hospital to home.* Springhouse, PA: Springhouse Corp.

Strassner, L. (1997). Critical pathways: The next generation of outcomes tracking. *Orthopaedic Nursing*, 16(2), S56. Retrieved June 27, 2003 from Infotrac database.

# CHAPTER 1c

# The Foundation of Outcome-Based Home Care: Outcomes Measurement and Standards of Care

# Patient Compliance: A Critical Role in Outcomes Management

| CORE TERMS AND CONCEPTS |
|---|
| • Patient compliance |
| • Compliance as an outcome |
| • Noncompliance as a variance |

## LEARNING OBJECTIVES

Upon completion of this topic, you will be able to:

1. Define patient compliance.
2. Recognize issues and circumstances that may negatively affect compliance.
3. List strategies that can help patients improve compliance.
4. Describe how patient compliance affects outcomes.
5. Describe how noncompliance can be tracked as a variance.
6. Describe how compliance can be measured as an outcome.

## AGENCY-SPECIFIC DATA/RESOURCES NEEDED

None

# INTRODUCTION

Clinicians have made judgments about patient compliance since home care's early beginnings. In the past, our judgments about a patient's compliance have been generally limited to documentation in the medical record as a pattern of behavior, brought to the physician's attention as appropriate to discuss continuation of services. However, because compliance has been determined as a key factor affecting outcomes (Cramer, 2002), complication rates (Osborne, 2002), and the cost of care, estimated at $100 billion for medication noncompliance alone (Walker, 2001), its role has come to the forefront in achieving desired outcomes.

Compliance not only affects outcomes, but it can also be measured as an outcome itself (Balon, 2002; Cramer, 2002; Kleinpell, 2001; Stone, Shiffman, Schwartz, Broderick, and Hufford, 2002). This section will explore both. We will examine the complexity of issues that affect compliance, the strategies to improve it, and discuss how compliance affects outcomes. We will discuss how compliance can be measured as an outcome or simply be tracked and aggregated as a variance in patient response to treatment.

## WHAT IS PATIENT COMPLIANCE?

Compliance has been defined as *the degree to which the patient follows health interventions as agreed with the health provider* (Cleemput and Kestlefoot, 2002; Cramer, 2002). Shifting the entire burden to the patient is no longer an option (Guglielmo, 2001). This definition recognizes both the provider and the patient as active participants in an acceptable compromise (Cherner, 2001; Walker, 2001). This compromise may include discussing the recommended treatment regimen and the patient's priorities, agreeing to modify dosing schedules whenever possible, and discussing lifestyle and cultural beliefs with respect to treatment modifications.

## FACTORS AFFECTING PATIENT COMPLIANCE

It is essential to determine the factors that affect compliance, because compliance affects healthcare outcomes. Compliance with treatment and medication regimens results in improved health status, enhanced lifestyle changes, decreased rates of hospitalization, increased healthful behaviors, lowering of disease risk, and improved patient satisfaction with care. Noncompliance is associated with higher risk of complications, increased hospitalizations, and increased healthcare costs (Cramer, 2002; Osborne, 2002; Walker, 2001).

The first step in managing compliance is to recognize factors that lead to noncompliance (Balon, 2002). Schechter and Walker (2002) found the risk of adherence to treatment to be essentially the same in all patient groups. While many of the studies regarding compliance have focused primarily on medications, other factors, as noted by Fawcett (1995), can have implications for treatment in general and are worthy of consideration in the planning and provision of care. These include:

- Patient characteristics
- Treatment setting
- Medications
- Clinical features of the illness
- Clinician expertise

Familiarize yourself with the guiding questions below and incorporate these into your initial patient assessment and the provision of care as appropriate to determine if issues that may affect the patient's compliance with his or her prescribed treatment regimen exist.

## Patient Characteristics—Guiding Questions

- What are the patient and caretaker's attitudes toward the condition or illness?
- Are there socioeconomic considerations that will restrict patient adherence to treatment?
- Is cost a factor?
- Will cultural beliefs affect recommended treatment regimens?
- Does the patient's ability to manage the condition require a certain amount of caretaker support? Is caretaker support available? If so, is the support coming from friends or family? Is this support dependable?
- Is the patient elderly? The prevalence of noncompliance in the elderly is high with common forms being medication overuse and abuse, forgetting, and alteration of doses and schedules (Salzman, 1995).
- What are the patient's attitudes about the medications that have been prescribed? Does the patient have any concern about taking the medicine that has been prescribed? Patients treated for a variety of medical disorders take on average approximately 75% of medications as prescribed, regardless of the potential for negative consequences (Cramer, 2002).
- What is the patient's tolerance level of pain? How does the patient feel about taking medication for pain? Is the patient expecting a great deal of pain with this condition based upon others' experiences? Is the patient more likely to try other methods of pain relief prior to taking prescribed medication?

## Treatment Setting

- Hospitals provide a setting where variables may be more easily controlled and compliance achieved because, due to the acuity of the illness, patients are in a more dependent state. For example, dietary choices are more controlled and nurses administer medications, except in cases where self-administration has been approved by policy.
- Home care provides a unique opportunity for clinicians in that they may see first-hand the issues that can affect the patient's compliance. For example, the clinician can see how medications are organized and stored and can offer suggestions as appropriate. Visual assessments of the home environment can be made and safety recommendations offered.
- Outpatient settings can offer support onsite that may be crucial for some patients. However, other outpatient services may present obstacles if travel or distance is an issue for the patient. For example, exercise programs that can be implemented at home may be more attractive to the patient who must depend on others for transportation or who live a prohibitive distance from the facility.

## Medications

- Clinicians face several challenges in helping patients manage medications. Each year 125,000 people die from some type of medication noncompliance; 10% of all hospitalizations and 14.5% of emergency department visits are attributed to prescription drug related problems (Walker, 2001).
- In Schechter and Walker's work with diabetic patients (2002), they state that self-reports of compliance are generally overestimated. Stone, Shiffman, Schwartz, Broderick, and Hufford (2002) documented that patients reported compliance to be 90%, while the actual was 11%. Williard and Olsen (2003) identify the five most common forms of medication noncompliance. These are:

  - Not having prescriptions filled
  - Taking the incorrect dose
  - Taking medicine at the wrong time

– Forgetting to take one or more doses
– Stopping the medicine too soon

Some questions that will be helpful in your assessment are:
• Have you filled your prescriptions? If the patient or caretaker has not, try to determine the reason.
• Are medications in appropriate containers and labeled correctly?
• Are there side effects that are annoying? Intolerable? Is the dosing schedule simple or complex? Cramer (2002) concluded that improved compliance rates are most associated with the number of doses to be taken daily, rather than the number of pills that must be taken.
• Is there a scheduling mechanism to manage multiple medications?
• Is the potential high for drug-drug or food-drug interactions?

## Clinical Features of the Illness

Certain features of conditions and types of illness have been found to have negative influences on patient compliance. Three of these are listed below:

1. Does the patient have a chronic condition? Patients with chronic illness have been shown to have only a 50% compliance rate with medications after one year (Barber, 2002), and further declines thereafter (Walker, 2001).
2. Are there co-morbid conditions that may complicate the patient's present condition? Co-morbid conditions generally result in more complex treatment regimens and often have more than one specialty physician treating the patient. The clinician's role as coordinator can have a positive impact on the patient's compliance.
3. Does the patient have a psychiatric illness? In psychiatric disorders, exaggerated feelings of one kind or another may present themselves in addition to the primary illness, making compliance difficult.

## Clinician Expertise

The health professional must recognize factors that affect compliance and work with the patient to minimize these. This requires knowledge of compliance issues, medical condition(s), and pharmacology. Knowing that adherence to treatment is improved through an understanding of the medication side effects, interactions, and precautions (Balon, 2002), clinicians must use their expertise to ensure that the patient/caretaker has a firm grasp of this subject matter. The clinician should keep in mind that information is best comprehended when presented in a format of basic to more complex concepts, and organize patient/caretaker teaching material and methods accordingly.

## STRATEGIES TO IMPROVE COMPLIANCE

There are four strategies that clinicians can use to help patients improve compliance and adherence to treatment. These are:

1. Patient self-management
2. Patient/caretaker education
3. Assistance with medication management
4. Effective communication and follow-up

## Patient Self-Management

Patient compliance is dramatically improved when a patient is self-assured and actively involved in his or her care (Cherner, 2001; Walker, 2001). Self-management has also been identified as critical for effective health promotion for successful home care of acute and chronic illness (Rice, 1998). One way of encouraging self-management is to first recognize the patient and caretaker's strengths.

During your admission assessment, pay particular attention to OASIS responses that give you a measure of the patient's cognition, function, emotion, and health status and that describe the home environment and support systems available to the patient. Correlate these findings with the skills the patient and caretaker need to manage the condition in the health provider's absence. For example, managing a moderately complex wound dressing may be too much for an older caretaker who has complete responsibility for managing the household, is the primary caretaker to the patient, and has arthritis and poor eyesight.

Another way of encouraging self-management is to ask open-ended questions and really listen to the patient/caretaker responses (Lyman, 2001). Knowing that patients judge treatment regimens according to social implications, such as where treatment interferes with the patient's *normalcy* (McPherson and Binning, 2002), clinicians can use information about the patient's lifestyle to gain insight into barriers that might not otherwise surface during the patient assessment. Explore these as appropriate, and often the solutions will become obvious.

For example, a patient with an artificial knee replacement has not been as compliant with his home exercise program as the therapist anticipated. The patient has continued pain. During a review of his medications, the clinician finds the bottle almost full and begins to ask more questions. The patient is concerned about becoming addicted because of an experience that a close family member had and has not taken the medicine as prescribed. The increased pain prevents the patient from achieving optimal flexion and extension in his home exercise program, which causes the affected limb to become stiff and more painful.

## Patient/Caretaker Education

A key element of successful education strategies is providing simple, clear messages, tailored to the individual and verifying that the messages have been understood (Gilford-Blake, 2002). Based upon your assessment, give information about the illness appropriate to the patient or caretaker's level of understanding, interest, and concern. Consider both the patient and primary caretaker(s) when deciding what type of teaching materials and methods to use. Will the caretaker be taking a great deal of responsibility for assisting the patient? Note the caretaker's capabilities of learning how to manage the illness. Is reading or writing the English language difficult for the patient and/or caretaker?

When the patient understands risks, benefits, and medical instructions, adherence rates tend to be significantly higher (Osborne, 2002). Explain the possible outcomes of the condition when prescribed treatment is not followed; for example, the cause and possible effect of a diabetic patient not inspecting his feet, the CHF patient not limiting sodium intake, or the orthopedic patient not abiding by weight bearing recommendations.

## Assistance with Medication Management

Teaching patients about medications is not new. However, what we know about medication compliance suggests that clinicians should routinely consider additional strategies to assist patients and caretakers to *manage* their medicines. Clinicians must acknowledge that the patient's agenda, not their own, determines whether he or she will take medicines as prescribed (Marinker and Shaw, 2003). A patient's own priorities and rationale have an impact upon adherence. Have prescriptions been filled? Costs or lack of transportation may be prohibiting factors, for which social services or the local pharmacist may be able to provide assistance.

Uncovering any preconceived notions, fears, misconceptions, or myths that the patient has about his or her condition or medications may be significant and should be addressed to the extent possible. Use a nonjudgmental approach of care and concern to make the patient or caretaker feel comfortable and free to express his or her thoughts. Assess both prescribed and over-the-counter medications not only for interactions, but also to determine if the patient is trying to achieve the same effect from over-the-counter medication due to prohibitive costs. Elicit the help of social services and the pharmacy.

Providing pill boxes and timing medications with personal rituals, such as brushing one's teeth, meal times, or tuning in to a favorite TV program to jog one's memory have been methods used by homecare nurses that work quite well. Given what we now know about compliance, consider a more simplified dosing schedule whenever possible. It is likely to enhance compliance even more (Bayliss, Park, Westfall, and Zamorski, 2001; Cramer, 2002). Consider fewer doses whenever possible. Discuss your thoughts with the patient's physician.

## Effective Communication and Follow-up

Cherner (2001) reports that patients tend to be more compliant when a reasonable compromise exists between clinician and patient. This requires that the clinician establish a good rapport and be willing to work within the patient's habits, lifestyle, and beliefs as much as possible. A partnering attitude toward patient and caretaker is recommended (Osborne, 2002). Osborne reported one study that found active collaboration between patient and provider not only improved compliance, but enhanced the patient's quality of life. Wachter (2003) recommends that clinicians be honest with patients and encourage their honesty, be empathetic to their concerns, invite questions, pick up on nonverbal cues, and accept a degree of noncompliance.

Keeping in touch with patients through telephone follow-up, e-mail reminders, and/or written notes results in greater participation in the treatment regimen (Schechter and Walker, 2002). Personal follow-up not only conveys a message of concern for the patient's well-being, but is also an opportunity for the clinician to solicit questions and to provide encouragement. Reminders to keep appointments (physician, home care visits, outpatient schedules) have also been found to be beneficial.

## ASSESSING COMPLIANCE

Whether you are making a subjective assessment about a patient's compliance with treatment or you have established a more quantitative measure, such as electronic monitoring of medication dosing, it is prudent to make an overall assessment of compliance as it relates to patient conditions and/or populations, or as it affects other outcomes. This information is used to improve care strategies and to market your services. For example, if national studies conclude that 50% of the patients with CHF admit noncompliance with medication and diet recommendations, the agency has a benchmark against which to compare these elements in their CHF patient population.

In another example, it is generally reported that only 50% of patients on long-term therapy actually take their medications as prescribed (Barber, 2002; Patients' failure to adhere, 2001; Walker, 2001). This information prompts an agency with a large number of hypertension patients to implement a special medication compliance program and to measure compliance as an outcome in this patient group. After six months, the agency's patients demonstrate a 70% compliance with their antihypertensive medications. This success can be shared with physician customers and other referral sources to recognize that significant improvements have been made with this patient group, and to evaluate if further improvements can be made.

An assessment of compliance can be accomplished through:

1. documenting, tracking, and aggregating *noncompliance* as a *variance* that affects outcomes, or
2. measuring and aggregating *compliance as an outcome* itself.

## Tracking Noncompliance as a Variance

Let's first examine noncompliance as a cause of *variance.* Noncompliance can be managed like other variances that are tracked through care pathways or other means of documentation. Once identified, it is typically addressed as a problem by the clinician, documented according to policy, and then entered into the agency's variance tracking system. Being tracked as a cause of variance, noncompliance is aggregated as a percentage to determine its overall presence in certain patient populations. This percentage is then evaluated retrospectively in relation to and in light of other patient discharge outcomes.

For example, an agency has noncompliance as a cause of variance for 68% of its CHF patients. The outcomes of this population are concurrently reviewed for one quarter and reveal that 48% of the patients experienced weight gain outside of acceptable limits and that the OASIS outcome of *Improvement in Dyspnea* is above the national reference mean. Given these percentages, you consider noncompliance as a likely factor in the weight gain and dyspnea. However, chart review must be conducted to make a more precise clinical judgment.

When noncompliance is tracked as a variance, be aware that you are tracking the *general existence* of noncompliance itself. Unless you design your care pathway or intervention sequence of events and variance tracking system to include *specific reasons* for noncompliance, the only conclusion you will be able to draw is that general noncompliance exists in a patient or patient group. Though general, this finding can still be useful in giving a sense of direction to performance improvement activities as demonstrated in the above example.

## Measuring Compliance as an Outcome

Compliance can be measured as an outcome itself (Balon, 2002; "Concordance and," 2003; Kleinpell, 2001) Clinicians make certain observations and are attentive to particular cues that result in judgments about patient compliance. Generally, if noncompliance exists, it is addressed to the extent possible, documented in the medical record, and communicated to the physician. This is at best a subjective measurement. Measuring or trying to quantify compliance is also largely subjective. As long as this is recognized and acknowledged, subjective compliance measurements are acceptable (R. Balon, personal communication, July 17, 2003).

Measuring compliance as an outcome allows an agency to determine when compliance is or is not achieved for certain elements of care. It affords the opportunity to extract compliance from the medical record and to aggregate it across patient populations or diagnoses. For example, measuring patient compliance with an exercise program or with keeping a timely food journal pinpoints specific areas where compliance is an issue. The advantage is that it facilitates more efficient and focused remediation efforts when outcomes are less than desired.

The most common clinical practice of measuring compliance is to ask patients to estimate their own level of compliance (Schechter and Walker, 2002). This can be accomplished by using structured self-report techniques of collecting data, the most common method used in nursing (Polit, Beck, and Hungler, 2001). These techniques may include response alternatives that range from a simple yes or no to complex expressions. Patient responses can be obtained during the course of each home visit or patient encounter and divided by the number of total visits or encounters to obtain a percentage of compliance or noncompliance for the patient (R. Balon, personal communication, July 17, 2003).

It is important to note that patient self-reporting tends to be overestimated. Schechter and Walker (2002) note several reasons for this:

- Patient reliance on memory or interpretation of the instructions given by clinicians
- The degree to which patients and caretakers follow instructions
- Trying to please the clinician
- Wanting to avoid embarrassment

Lower estimates of compliance are typically found when measures such as pill counts, completeness of food diaries, and monitoring logs are used (Schechter and Walker, 2002).

Efforts are being made to establish more objective types of compliance measurements. Some of these include: electronic monitoring devices, prescription counting or pill counts, and biological measurements, such as drug levels, assays, and weight gain or loss.

---

### CONCEPT APPLICATION:
### Ascertaining Patient Compliance

An agency measures the following compliance outcome indicators for all patients with a primary diagnosis of diabetes who are insulin dependent:

*Patient is compliant with special diet, and*
*Patient is compliant with maintaining a daily, current finger stick glucose log.*

The agency decides to collect compliance data from the patient or caretaker each visit. The clinician first asks general open-ended questions about the patient's adjustment to the diet since the last visit. The clinician then asks the patient if he or she was able to stay within the special diet guidelines since this time and if any obstacles were met, such as food preparation or purchase and remembering to eat or not to eat certain foods. A simple yes or no is noted. The agency decides that the clinician will enter a "No" response if the patient or caretaker reports that the patient did not comply with the special diet at any time.

Also, the finger stick glucose log is reviewed with the patient to determine if entries are up to date. The clinician makes another yes or no notation of whether the patient was compliant with this self-management skill by observing all log entries made since the last visit.

At the end of the episode, responses are aggregated for the patient as a whole. "Yes" responses are totaled for each compliance indicator and divided by the number of visits during which responses were ascertained. This simple proportion is expressed as a percentage for the group (Motulsky, 1995). "Yes" responses can be aggregated to note compliance or "No" responses can be aggregated to note noncompliance.

At the end of each quarter, responses for these two compliance outcome indicators are aggregated for this patient group discharged during the quarter. The findings reveal that 67% of these patients report that they are adhering to the special diet and 72% are compliant with maintaining a current glucose log. The agency sets its own thresholds for acceptable percentages according to its quality of care issues, performance improvement goals, or business strategy.

The agency reviews these compliance outcomes relative to its OASIS Adverse Event Outcome percentage of Emergent care for hypo/hyperglycemia, which is higher than the national reference. The agency wants to know if there is a correlation between compliance with the diet, maintaining a current finger stick log and Emergent care for hypo/hyperglycemia. Further investigation and chart review is needed however, to draw this conclusion.

## AGENCY APPLICATION:
## Measuring Individual Patient Compliance

Clinicians assess the following compliance outcome indicator for every patient who has a primary diagnosis of hypertension:

*Patient is compliant with obtaining or performing daily BP checks.*

Each clinician enters a "yes" or "no" response each visit within the agency's documentation format indicating the patient's compliance with this self management skill.

The patient has nine visits over the course of an episode.

Patient responses for compliance are:  Yes–Yes–Yes–No–Yes–Yes–No–Yes–Yes

Calculate a percentage of the time that this patient reported compliance:

Number of "Yes" responses _____ (divided by) the total number of compliance responses _____ = _____% compliance with the self-management skill.

*Answer: 7 "Yes" responses (divided by) 9 total compliance responses = 77 % self-reported compliance*

## AGGREGATION OF COMPLIANCE PERCENTAGES

Aggregation of compliance percentages can be calculated for a patient population or group. However, keep in mind that the smaller the population the less significant or meaningful the findings become (M.A. Smith, personal communication, February 18, 2004). Averages across larger populations have greater meaning.

A baseline threshold percentage is selected that the agency feels is reasonable and realistic to achieve. The aggregation percentage for the patient group is evaluated and compared to this threshold. Performance improvement efforts may be initiated to determine why a percentage is below the agency's threshold.

Aggregation can be performed manually or via automation. Automation is by far the most efficient. Your agency's software program can be written to calculate compliance outcome percentages for your patient population(s) or groups and to provide this information in report form. A compliance aggregation report should at least include the following information:

*Compliance indicator*     *% Compliant or % Noncompliant*     *Agency Threshold %*

## AGENCY APPLICATION:
### Aggregating Patient Compliance

An agency ascertains an average percentage of self-reported compliance for twenty hypertensive patients discharged in the second quarter. The compliance outcome is:

*Patient is compliant with obtaining or performing daily BP checks.*

| Patient Compliance Percentage | Number of Patients |
|---|---|
| 77% | 2 |
| 79% | 2 |
| 80% | 3 |
| 81% | 4 |
| 83% | 2 |
| 85% | 1 |
| 86% | 1 |
| 92% | 3 |
| 100% | 2 |

1. Obtain the average percentage of self-reported compliance for this patient group.

   Total of Percentages _____ (divided by) Total # of patients _____

   = _____ % self-reported compliance for this patient group.

*Answer: 1689 / 20 = This patient group has 84% self-reported compliance with obtaining or performing daily BP checks.*

2. Using your agency's performance improvement goals, select a percentage threshold that you consider satisfactory for this compliance indicator for the patient population in question.  *Note: It may take more than one quarter to establish a reasonable and realistic baseline agency threshold.

## Guiding Questions

- Is the agency compliance threshold percentage reasonable and realistic for the patient population in question?

- Are compliance outcome indicators appropriate to skills and information learned by the patient or caretaker?

- Does enough time remain on service for the patient or caretaker to comply with skills and information learned?

## USING COMPLIANCE IN OUTCOMES ANALYSIS

Measuring or tracking compliance gives helpful insight and perspective to other outcomes achieved. When analyzing *outcomes* that *are less than desired*, your investigation should start with the questions, "Why?", "Did we teach the patient the right things?", "Did we provide care according to our agency standards of care?" If this answer is yes, the next question is "Did the patient/caretaker adhere to treatment regimens and comply with doing the things that were taught?" An agency can do a great job of teaching self-care management skills to the patient/caretaker only to discover that noncompliance has affected other outcomes adversely.

For example, an agency evaluates the OASIS outcome: *Improvement in dsypnea* and its own supplemental outcome of: Patient/caregiver demonstrates safe and proper use of oxygen and equipment.

Not only does the patient with COPD not progress, but he worsens in the OASIS outcome and has to seek emergent care during the length of service. However, the patient achieves the outcome of being able to demonstrate safe and proper use of oxygen and equipment. The information you have is valuable; the patient worsened, yet he knew how to manage his oxygen and equipment. You can eliminate lack of proper management of oxygen and equipment as the cause.

While there are other clinical and educational outcomes that your agency has measured related to COPD, you have no readily available information in reference to the patient's compliance with treatment and how this has affected the outcomes. A compliance outcome in this case can help you quickly eliminate noncompliance as the cause and allow you to focus your investigation elsewhere.

## DEVELOPING MEASURABLE COMPLIANCE OUTCOME INDICATORS

When deciding which compliance outcome indicators to measure, first **consider the educational outcomes** that you have written. Secondly, note the **applicability of compliance** as it relates to these same educational outcomes. Thirdly, **evaluate the appropriateness** of the compliance outcomes you have in mind. Fourthly, **consider compliance** as it relates to the **primary diagnoses** that comprise your greatest volume, that are the most problematic, or that have important relevance to agency goals.

For example, the outcome *Patient compliant with a home exercise program* **is applicable** in that your therapists are teaching the patient a home exercise program that he or she is to perform four times a week. Noncompliance with the program may adversely affect the patient's functional status resulting in slower recovery, possible complications, and increased costs. In this case, measuring compliance **is appropriate** in that it is reasonable to determine if the patient is performing the exercises as instructed.

In addition to the sessions with the therapist, the patient may be required to perform the exercises independently, making it important to know if the patient is adhering to the rehabilitation prescription. It would not be appropriate to measure the patient's *compliance with verbalizing the components of the exercise program* because there is nothing regarding *verbalization of the program* for the patient to comply with. The patient either verbalizes the components or does not.

Measuring this compliance outcome is also important to the agency because total knee replacement is its **number three diagnosis** in volume in the last year, and it has entered into an alliance with a local hospital to provide the continuation of a specialty rehabilitation program that begins as an inpatient.

## AGENCY APPLICATION:
### Writing Compliance Outcome Indicators

Consider the following outcome indicators for the patient with CHF:

OASIS outcome:
1. *Improvement in dyspnea*

Agency supplemental outcome indicators:

1. Patient/caretaker verbalizes adverse signs and symptoms to report by visit two.
2. Patient/caretaker demonstrates proper method of weighing self daily by visit three.
3. Patient/caretaker verbalizes importance of low sodium intake by visit five.

Write two compliance outcomes for the patient with CHF that are *relative to the knowledge outcomes above.*

1. _____

2. _____


Consider the following outcome indicators for the patient with a pressure ulcer:

OASIS outcomes:
1. *Increase in number of pressure ulcers*
2. *Emergent care for wound infections, deteriorating wound status*

Agency supplemental outcome indicators:

1. Patient/caretaker demonstrates ability to properly reduce pressure by visit three.
2. Patient/caretaker verbalizes importance of protein and calories for healing by visit six.
3. Patient/caretaker demonstrates proper wound cleansing and dressing application by visit seven.
4. Patient/caretaker verbalizes adverse signs and symptoms of wound infection and deterioration by visit eight.


Write two compliance outcome indicators for a patient/caretaker managing a pressure ulcer that are *relative to the knowledge outcomes preceding.*

1. _____

2. _____

**AGENCY APPLICATION:**

**Writing Compliance Outcome Indicators** *(continued)*

Consider the following outcome indicators for the patient with tuberculosis (TB):

OASIS outcomes: *Not applicable here for TB.*

Agency supplemental outcome indicators:

1. Patient/caretaker verbalizes the disease process by visit two.
2. Patient/caretaker demonstrates proper infection control measures by visit three.
3. Patient/caretaker verbalizes TB medication dose, actions, precautions, side effects, and dosing schedule by visit five.
4. Patient/caretaker demonstrates energy conservation measures by visit six.

Write a compliance outcome indicator for a patient who has TB.

_____

_____

_____

_____

_____

_____

1c

## REFERENCES

Balon, R. (2002). Managing compliance. *Biomechanics*, May 1, p. 43. Retrieved June 27, 2003 from Infotrac database.

Barber, N. (2002). Should we consider non-compliance a medical error? *Quality and Safety in Healthcare*, 11(1), 81. Retrieved June 27, 2003 from Infotrac database.

Bayliss, E. A., Park, M. K., Westfall, J. M., & Zamorski, M. A. (2001). How can I improve patient adherence to prescribed medication? *Journal of Family Practice*, 50(4), 303. Retrieved June 27, 2003 from Infotrac database.

Cherner, R. (2001). Diabetes therapy: How to enlist patient compliance. *Consultant*, 41(9), 1259. Retrieved June 27, 2003 from Infotrac database.

Cleemput, I. & Kestefoot, K. (2002). Economic implications of non-compliance in health care. *The Lancet*, 359(9324), 2129. Retrieved June 27, 2003 from Infotrac database.

Concordance and compliance. (2003). *Thorax*, 58(2), 59. Retrieved June 27, from Infotrac database.

Cramer, J. A. (2002). Effect of partial compliance on cardiovascular medication effectiveness. *Heart*, 88(2), 203. Retrieved June 27, 2003 from Infotrac database.

Fawcett, J. (1995). Compliance: Definitions and key issues. *Journal of Clinical Psychiatry*, 56 (supp 1), 4–8. Retrieved June 27, 2003 from Infotrac database.

Gilford-Blake, R. (2002). Communication critical to management of chronic conditions in the elderly. *Managedhealthcare. Info*, August 5, p. 4. Retrieved June 27, 2003 from Infotrac database.

Guglielmo, W. J. (2001). Follow-up care: Nuts, bolts, carrots, and sticks. *Medical Economics*, 78(18), 30. Retrieved June 27, 2003 from Infotrac database.

Kleinpell, R. M. (Ed.). (2001). *Outcome assessment in advanced practice*. NY: Springer Publishing Co.

Lyman, G. (2001). Getting patients to follow through on treatment plans. *Healthcare Review*, 14(4), 29. Retrieved June 27, 2003 from Infotrac database.

McPherson, M. V. & Binning, J. (2002). Chronic foot ulcers associated with diabetes: Patients' views. *The Diabetic Foot*, 5(4), 198. Retrieved June 27, 2003 from Infotrac database.

Marinker, M. & Shaw, J. (2003). Not to be taken as directed: Putting concordance for taking medicines into practice. *British Medical Journal*, 326(7385), 348. Retrieved June 27, 2003 from Infotrac database.

Motulsky, H. (1995). *Intuitive biostatistics*. Oxford, England: Oxford University Press, Inc.

Osborne, H. (2002). The value of partnering with patients. *Health Care, Food & Nutrition Focus*, 18(11), 1.

Patients' failure to adhere to prescriptions accounts for 10% of hospital admissions. (2001). *Health Care Strategic Management*, 19(6), 10. Retrieved June 27, 2003 from Infotrac database.

Polit, D. F., Beck, C. T., & Hungler, B. P. (2001). *Essentials of nursing research: Methods, appraisal and utilization*. Philadelphia: Lippincott.

Rice, R. (1998). Key concepts of self-care in the home: Implications for home care nurses. *Geriatric Nursing*, 19(1), 52–54.

Salzman, C. (1995). Medication compliance in the elderly. *Journal of Clinical Psychiatry*, 56 (suppl 1), 18–22. Retrieved June 27, 2003 from Infotrac database.

Schechter, C. B. & Walker, E. A. (2002). Improving adherence to diabetes self-management recommendations. *Diabetes Spectrum*, 15(3), 170. Retrieved June 27, 2003 from Infotrac database.

Stone, A. A., Shiffman, S., Schwartz, J.E., Broderick, J. E., & Hufford, M. R. (2002). Patient non-compliance with paper diaries. *British Medical Journal*, 324(7347), 1193. Retrieved June 27, 2003 from Infotrac database.

Wachter, K. (2003). Work with patients is the key to improving medication adherence. *Clinical Psychiatry News*, 31(3), 18. Retrieved June 27, 2003 from Infotrac database.

Walker, T. (2001). Understanding patient needs is key to medication compliance. *Managed Healthcare Executive*, 11(1), 34. Retrieved June 27, 2003 from Infotrac database.

Williard, R. & Olsen, S. (2003). Congestive heart failure compliance. Retrieved July 22, 2003 from http://www.wwmr.com/eppub/cpc_v3.pdf.

# CHAPTER 1D

# The Foundation of Outcome-Based Home Care: Outcomes Measurement and Standards of Care

# Standards of Care/ Best Practices

---

**LEARNING OBJECTIVES**

Upon completion of this topic, you will be able to:

1. Define a standard of care/best practices.
2. Describe the difference in providing a standard of care versus usual care.
3. Describe how standards of care are developed.
4. Formulate standards of care pertinent to patients served.
5. Explain the use of patient teaching materials as a standard of care.

---

**CORE TERMS AND CONCEPTS**

- Standards of Care
- Clinical Practice Guideline
- Evidence-Based Practice
- Best Practices
- Usual Care

---

**AGENCY-SPECIFIC DATA/RESOURCES NEEDED**

- Access to the Internet
- Agency's current patient teaching material for pressure ulcer prevention

# INTRODUCTION

Outcome-based patient care depends on outcomes achieved and the clinical interventions that help achieve them. There are interventions that are more likely to produce certain outcomes than others. This reflects a relationship between interventions provided and outcomes achieved. It is this relationship that prompts health professionals to continually seek to improve clinical interventions in hopes of improving patient outcomes.

This section examines different types of clinical interventions and shows you how to determine which ones are likely to achieve desired outcomes. It distinguishes standards of care from usual care and discusses the application of best practices.

## WHAT IS A STANDARD OF CARE?

A standard is defined as *a rule or principle established by authority to measure quality or value* (Merriam-Webster, 2002). Standards of care typically reflect guidelines (*principles*) that are set up (*established*) by those in authority (*state boards governing clinical practice, federal government, organizations, and agency management*) as a measure (*yardstick*) by which quality (*practice*) is gauged.

Clinicians consider the individual patient circumstance and then implement a standard of care for each patient who has the problem for which the standard applies (Humphrey and Malone-Nuzzo, 1996; Powell, 2001). An intervention in a standard of care may not be applicable to a particular patient, but the standard is generally applicable for all patients to which the standard applies.

For example, an agency adopts a standard of care for the patient with COPD that includes teaching energy conservation, breathing techniques, medication management, safety with oxygen and equipment, and a pulmonary rehabilitation program. The patient has an end-stage deteriorating condition, and the physician feels that rehabilitation is not appropriate at this time. The pulmonary rehabilitation program in this case is *not applicable* to the patient and is excluded from the standard interventions that are provided by staff. The other interventions in this agency's standard of care are provided to the patient.

## STANDARD OF CARE VERSUS USUAL CARE

A standard of care differs from usual care in that *usual care is directed by medical orders and varies in its implementation from clinician to clinician* (Tinetti, Baker, Gallo, Nanda, Charpentier, and O'Leary, 2002). The following example shows the contrast between implementing a standard of care and providing usual care:

A patient has a primary diagnosis of hypertension. The physician orders the blood pressure to be taken every visit and for the staff to teach hypertension risk management to the patient and caretaker.

### Providing Usual Care

- Each nurse uses clinical judgment during the home visit to determine if blood pressure readings need to be taken while the patient is sitting only, sitting and standing, or sitting, standing, and lying.
- Each clinician selects patient education material of his or her choice from which to teach hypertension management and risk reduction.

### Implementing a Standard of Care

An excerpt from a standard of care at Agency ABC states that:
All patients with a primary diagnosis of hypertension will:

- have blood pressure checked every visit while they are in a sitting, standing, and lying position.
- be taught hypertension management and risk reduction from XYZ Hypertension teaching booklet.

Every skilled nurse follows this standard every visit for every patient with a primary diagnosis of hypertension. *Exception*: A patient has dyspnea and cannot lie down to have his blood pressure checked in this position as the standard calls for. Taking the blood pressure while the patient is lying down is an intervention that is *not applicable* for this patient and is omitted from the standard of care in this circumstance.

**1**D

---

## CONCEPT APPLICATION:
### Identifying Standards of Care

Identify the statements below that reflect the implementation of a *standard of care* by writing **yes** in the blank provided.

_____ 1. Pressure ulcer risk assessment tool is completed for all adult patient admissions.

_____ 2. Physical therapists implement patient treatment plans for CVA according to their individual choice.

_____ 3. All patients with a vascular access device are taught to assess the site for redness, swelling, and drainage.

_____ 4. An agency's procedure for the neurological/circulatory assessment of a fractured extremity includes capillary refill, temperature, sensation, movement, and color.

_____ 5. An agency develops a CVA rehabilitation program with certain interventions planned for all patients entering the program.

Answers: *1, 3, 4, and 5*
Rationale: *Statement #2 reflects usual care; the clinician has own choice.*

---

## CONCEPT APPLICATION:
### Developing Standards of Care

An agency has patients with pressure ulcers who have longer lengths of stay compared to the company's benchmark average. It is determined that one area of concern is pressure reduction. The agency has compared the use of ABC patient turning schedule to another. The ABC schedule is easier for the caretaker to understand and comply with. Caretakers using this turning schedule report greater satisfaction with its use. The agency decides to include the use of this turning schedule in its standard of care for patients who have a primary or secondary diagnosis of pressure ulcer and for those identified at risk.

The *standard of care* is formulated into the following statement: All patients admitted with a primary or secondary diagnosis of pressure ulcer or who have been identified at risk for pressure ulcers by a score of "X" on the risk assessment tool are taught the use of the ABC patient turning schedule.

# WHAT ARE BEST PRACTICES?

Best practices are *optimal techniques, procedures, or programs identified through evidence-based research or field experience of one or more organizations* (Shears, 2003) that improve care effectiveness and efficiency while enhancing positive patient outcomes (Benefield, 2002). The term best practice is also frequently used as an umbrella label for algorithms, protocols, care pathways, and clinical practice guidelines that reflect optimal clinical interventions. The implementation of best practice is encouraged in patient care (Grol and Grimshaw, 2003) and is typically available in health literature.

In OBQI, the term best practices is used to denote *specific statements of clinical actions expected of staff in order to impact the problem or strength identified in the statement* (CMS, 2002). These statements can be based on scientific evidence, health literature, and/or PI findings. (*\*Note: The term **best practice interventions** is used throughout the workbook to denote clinical interventions that are considered best practice according to the health literature or OBQI.*)

The first logical step in developing standards of care in your agency is to review and evaluate existing best practices in the health literature. Best practices are made available to health professionals through clinical practice guidelines, evidence reports, and evidence summaries. These are collectively referred to as *evidence-based practice*.

## Evidence-Based Practice

Evidence-based practice is *using the best scientific evidence available to guide decision making* (Benefield, 2002). It is developed from the accumulation of a large body of studies (Stevens, 2002). Evidence for clinical decision making can be found in clinical practice guidelines, evidence reports, and evidence summaries that provide a review and analysis of conducted research (Stevens, 2002). The strength of evidence, sometimes called the level of recommendation for use (Stetler, 2001), ranks the strength and quality of the study findings (Benefield, 2002). If strengths of evidence are provided in the literature you are reviewing, a key is generally provided that identifies the rankings used. Rankings are provided as I, II, III, etc., or A, B, C, etc.

For example, an agency's OASIS outcomes of *Improvement in ambulation* and *Improvement in transfer* are somewhat lower than the national reference mean and meet OBQI criteria as target outcomes. After investigating possible reasons and considering the age of its patient population, the agency director contacts physical therapists and physical therapy assistants who provide therapy services on an individual contract basis. They meet with nursing managers and decide to develop a standard of care using information from the National Institute on Aging (NIA) and the National Arthritis Foundation (NAF), both of whom base their recommendations on medical research (NIA, 2003; NAF, 2003). Strength of evidence is provided. The agency's medical director provides additional input.

Agency representatives develop a patient teaching handout for improving mobility based upon the recommendations provided by these two nationally recognized groups. The nursing and therapy staffs agree that patients 70 years and older should receive this handout as a courtesy, and that patients 70 years and older, with OASIS responses of 2, 3, or 4, for items *M0690: Transferring* and *M0700: Ambulation and Locomotion* (CMS, 2002), should be considered for therapy evaluation. Patients who are appropriate for therapy treatment receive additional instruction that includes information as appropriate from the handout. The agency uses these recommendations to develop a *standard of care* for this patient group.

In a second example, an agency is developing a care pathway for the care of cardiac surgical patients. The development team wants to include a psychosocial category on the pathway. They review several research studies on the topic of psycho-education programs and their effect on the reduction of cardiac risk factors, cardiac mortality, and recurrent MI. These studies show that patients who attended these programs had better outcomes (Fonteyn, 2002).

The agency uses these findings to develop its standards of care for the psychosocial element of the pathway (Gingerich and Ondeck, 2000). It includes information to help the patient and caretaker/spouse deal with fear and anxiety and to recognize and report early signs and symptoms of depression.

## Clinical Practice Guidelines

1D

These guidelines are *systematically developed statements based on scientific methodology and expert clinical judgment that assist in practitioner and patient decisions about health care for certain clinical conditions* (DHHS, 1995). A clinical practice guideline outlines best practice interventions that should be considered for implementation in most circumstances, with professional judgment making the final determination (Powell, 2001). Clinical/practice guidelines are used as one method to improve patient outcomes (Goode et al., 2000).

For example, the Agency for Healthcare Research and Quality (AHRQ) has a clinical practice guideline containing best practice interventions for the prevention of pressure ulcers in adults (DHHS, 1992). These interventions include:

- Risk assessment
- Skin care and early treatment
- Mechanical loading and support surfaces
- Education

An agency uses this guideline to develop a standard of care for the prevention of pressure ulcers. Senior clinicians and management staff review the clinical practice guideline and consider these recommendations in light of care currently provided by the agency. One of the AHRQ's recommendations is the periodic use of a valid risk assessment tool to identify patients at risk for the development of pressure ulcers. Currently the agency does not require the use of a specific risk assessment tool.

The AHRQ guideline gives examples of assessment tools that meet its criteria. The agency must ask:

- Which risk assessment tool will we use?
- How often will patients be assessed for risk?
- Who will complete the risk assessment?
- Will it be used for every patient or selected patients?

The agency selects a valid risk assessment tool to be used by physical therapists and registered nurses during the admission and recertification of all adult patients. This becomes an agency *standard of care*.

## CONCEPT APPLICATION:
### Locating Clinical Practice Guidelines

*Note: The National Guidelines Clearinghouse, developed by the Agency for Healthcare Research and Quality in partnership with the American Medical Association and the American Association of Health Plans, is the Internet repository for clinical practice guidelines (Benefield, 2002). The individual taskforces who formulate these guidelines update them periodically.*

1. Access the Internet.

2. Enter the following web address: http://www.guideline.gov.

3. Scroll through the sets of guidelines to familiarize yourself with the listing.

4. Scroll to Agency for Healthcare Research and Quality.

5. Locate the guideline for pressure ulcer prevention and treatment.

6. Review the guideline.

7. Scroll to the Wound, Ostomy, and Continence Nurse Society.

8. Review the guideline for pressure ulcers.

9. Notice similarities and differences in the two guidelines.

10. Print the AHRQ guideline.

## AGENCY APPLICATION:
### Evaluating a Clinical Practice Guideline for Agency Use

This application guides you through the evaluation of each intervention in a clinical practice guideline for applicability to your patient populations.

1. Refer to your copy of the AHRQ's clinical practice guideline for pressure ulcer prevention for more detail.

2. Review each intervention in the guideline.

3. Compare these recommendations to your agency's current practice.

4. Note the similarities and differences.

1D

## AGENCY APPLICATION:

### Evaluating a Clinical Practice Guideline for Agency Use
*(continued)*

Beside each element below, write "yes" if your agency currently includes this intervention or "no" if your agency does not include the intervention in the prevention of pressure ulcers.

- **Risk assessment**
  - _____ Use of a valid risk assessment tool
  - _____ Periodic use of
- **Skin care and early treatment**
  - _____ Skin inspection
  - _____ Skin cleansing
  - _____ Avoiding dry skin
  - _____ Massage
  - _____ Exposure to moisture
  - _____ Friction and shear injuries
  - _____ Nutrition
  - _____ Mobility/activity
- **Loading and support surface**
  - _____ Repositioning
  - _____ Positioning devices
  - _____ Pressure relief for heels
  - _____ Side lying positions
  - _____ Lifting devices
  - _____ Pressure reducing devices for beds
  - _____ Pressure from sitting
  - _____ Pressure reducing devices for chairs
  - _____ Postural alignment
- **Education topics for patients and staff**
  - _____ Etiology
  - _____ Risk assessment
  - _____ Skin assessment & care
  - _____ Selection & use of support surfaces
  - _____ Positioning

## Evidence Reports and Summaries

An evidence report *delineates how evidence-based practice is used in the clinical area* by providing an analysis of the scientific data, level of evidence, and recommendations for clinical practice (Benefield, 2002). This report rates the strength and quality of the study findings (DHHS, 2003).

An evidence summary or review provides an *analysis of the findings of multiple research studies and presents a state of the science conclusion* (Stevens, 2002). This summary typically includes variations of study findings and contradictory conclusions.

## IMPLEMENTING EVIDENCE-BASED PRACTICE

While it is ideal to provide evidence-based interventions to every patient for whom they are applicable, not all will be practical, reasonable, financially feasible, or appropriate for use in a particular agency setting. This is a decision the agency must make. How does the agency decide?

*Guiding Questions*

- Does the strength of the evidence support a change in agency practice?
- What is the benefit of interventions versus the risk to patients without them?
- Does the volume of patients with a particular diagnosis justify a change in existing practice?
- Are the changes in practice reasonable for our setting?
- Are interventions cost-effective? Can the agency afford to make changes to interventions? Can it afford not to?
- Is it feasible to implement these changes in our practice setting?

## OBQI BEST PRACTICES

OBQI best practices must be patient-care centered and reflect activities that are within an agency's control (CMS, 2002). For example, through OBQI activities, an agency finds that its outcome percentage of patients with urinary incontinence is above the national reference average. Patients receive usual care.

After chart review and staff interview, the agency decides to assess the need to initiate a formal bladder training program as part of the care provided to all patients, with a primary or secondary diagnosis of urinary incontinence in hopes of improving this outcome.

A best practice statement written and adopted for use by the agency is: nursing staff will assess all adult patients admitted with a primary or secondary diagnosis of incontinence for the appropriateness of the agency's bladder training program. This becomes a standard of care for the agency.

In a second example, an agency performs an investigation of the OASIS adverse event outcome, *Emergent care for hypo/hyperglycemia*. The findings reveal two things that the majority of patients requiring emergent care have in common:

1. noncompliance with diet, as documented in the medical record
2. new diagnosis of insulin-dependent diabetes

Other findings indicate that usual care is provided to diabetics, dietary instruction is limited in scope and focus, and that continuity of care among nursing staff can be improved. The agency seeks the assistance of the local hospital's dietitian, who evaluates the various teaching materials used by staff. She also agrees to provide updated education periodically to staff and to make PRN visits for patients with newly diagnosed diabetes. The following becomes a standard of care for the agency:

All patients with newly diagnosed diabetes will:

1. Have at least one visit from a dietitian or certified diabetic educator during the first two weeks of service.
2. Receive diabetes instruction using the XYZ Diabetes teaching material throughout the length of service.

## WRITING AND IMPLEMENTING STANDARDS OF CARE

When writing a standard of care, stay focused on its purpose—to achieve an improved quality of care as measured by corresponding outcomes. To clarify specifics of the standard and its implementation, express the standard in sentence form.

For example, consider *risk assessment*, one area of recommendation in the clinical practice guideline for the prevention of pressure ulcers (DHHS, 2000). Risk assessment helps achieve a lower incidence of pressure ulcers in adults (DHHS, 2000). With this outcome in mind, Agency B writes the following standard of care for risk assessment to be implemented by clinicians: all adult patients are assessed for pressure ulcer risk on admission and at resumption of care and other follow-up, using the XYZ risk assessment tool.

While this statement may be used in policy or procedure as written, standards that are integrated into clinical practice do not always appear in long sentence form. For example, an agency revises its clinical forms to include a wound assessment reflective of the elements within the clinical practice guideline. The clinician is instructed to complete the form on every visit. The standard of care for wound assessment is reflected within the assessment itself.

Let's examine additional standards of care written by Agency B to *treat pressure ulcers* in adult patients. The outcomes the agency wants to achieve are:

- No increase in the number of pressure ulcers.
- No wound deterioration or infection post home care admission.

The clinical practice guideline is again reviewed for recommendations in light of the agency's patient population. An excerpt from the recommendations for the assessment of pressure ulcers (DHHS, 2000) includes the following:

- Determine the location, stage, and size of the pressure ulcer.
- Determine the presence of undermining, tunneling exudates, necrotic tissue, granulation, and epithelialization.
- Assess pressure ulcer at least once a week.
- If there is no evidence of healing, re-evaluate the plan after two-to-four weeks of initiation of treatment.

Based upon the outcomes the agency desires and the recommendations from an evidence-based clinical practice guideline, Agency B writes the following standards of care (excerpt only):

- Pressure ulcers are assessed and described during each dressing change and at least weekly to include location, stage, and size.
- Each pressure ulcer is photographed at least monthly. The photo becomes a part of the medical record and includes last name, date, and affected body part.
- Patient's consent for photographs is obtained prior to first picture taken.
- Ulcer(s) are measured weekly, using XYZ measuring device.
- Documentation of the measurement is length by width by depth.
- Assessment includes the presence or absence of undermining, tunneling, exudates, necrotic tissue, granulation, and epithelialization.
- If no evidence of healing is noted after two-to-four weeks of treatment, the agency manager is notified. Re-evaluation of and adherence to the plan is conducted. Physician is notified accordingly.

To implement these standards of care, the agency:

- Conducts staff education related to all aspects of the change, including why the standard is being implemented, how implementation will take place, and who will be affected by the change.
- Conducts staff competency assessments as needed.
- Re-designs the admission assessment and visit note to include recommended assessment items. Printed within the clinical note is the directive: *Measure ulcer on the first visit of each week. Describe every visit.*
- Clerk to place a *Consent to Photograph* form in the admission packet of patients whose referral to home care includes a diagnosis of pressure ulcer. New diagnosis

NOTES

1D

of pressure ulcer post admission requires completion of the form. Office staff performs a *check and balance* of this process. Auditing of clinical forms includes notation of the presence of completed form.

- Assures that XYZ wound measuring devices are readily available to clinicians and are stocked by the supply clerk. The measuring device has length by width by depth noted on it.
- Performs clinical data audits. During the first three months of implementation and periodically thereafter, a senior clinician reviews documentation to determine if time frames for assessing and measuring are being met and if documentation is complete according to the standard.

Note how each element in the standard aligns with the recommendations of the clinical practice guideline. Also note how implementation is planned to achieve maximum staff compliance with the standard. This includes incorporating new processes within the daily routines of care and addressing additional needs of documentation.

---

## AGENCY APPLICATION:
### Identifying Current Agency Standards

According to definition, identify any standard(s) of care that your agency currently implements for patients with a primary diagnosis of:

**Pressure Ulcer:**

_____

_____

_____

**Urinary Incontinence:**

_____

_____

_____

**Diabetes:**

_____

_____

_____

## PATIENT/CARETAKER EDUCATIONAL MATERIAL AS A STANDARD OF CARE

Homecare providers have long recognized that patient and family/caretaker education is a cornerstone in the provision of care. However, it has taken on additional meaning in a prospective pay environment. Self-care management has been identified as critical for effective health promotion for successful home health care of acute and chronic conditions (Rice, 1998).

These skills are used by patients and caretakers to attain, maintain, and promote wellness, as well as to promptly recognize and report untoward signs and symptoms. As the patient and caretaker assume a greater role in managing the patient's illness or condition, they have a greater need for the knowledge to manage it.

Using standardized patient teaching materials in appropriate situations affords us the opportunity to communicate and teach a standard of care, to enhance staff continuity of care, and to help focus patient and caretaker attention on the same subject matter, regardless of the clinician teaching it. In other words, the teaching material itself not only reflects the standards of care provided, but it also becomes a standard of care itself.

When developing patient teaching materials, make sure that the contents align with the standards of care you have written. For example, when teaching patients and caretakers how to inspect and assess bony prominences for redness, include basically the same information that is in your standard—the same used by agency clinicians to inspect and assess for redness. Provide this information at a third or fourth grade level for easy understanding, and provide it in written form for those who have no difficulty reading and writing at this level.

While this may seem obvious, it is not uncommon to see clinicians using different methods of assessing and different materials to teach the patient the same subject matter. The patient then has several viewpoints to sort through or may have only received one aspect of the subject matter repeatedly, with other important details omitted altogether.

The agency may use pre-printed materials provided by various national associations, organizations, and/or companies, or they can produce their own. They can also use a combination of both. When selecting pre-printed material, make sure that the information is in accordance with your standards of care.

**1**D

## AGENCY APPLICATION:
### Preparing Teaching Material as a Standard of Care

Refer to the AHRQ clinical practice guideline for the prevention of pressure ulcers.

- Review the items recommended for patient education.

- List specific elements in the guideline for patient education that are appropriate for your agency to consider in preparing standardized teaching material for this patient group:

1. _____

2. _____

3. _____

4. _____

5. _____

6. _____

7. _____

8. _____

9. _____

10. _____

### Guiding Questions

- Do the clinical practice guidelines you have located contain recommendations for patient education?

- Are there other resources available?

- Does the educational information already exist in a format suitable for patient learning?

- If so, do materials contain the standards of care that the agency wants/needs to provide?

- Will the agency develop its own teaching materials?

- If so, who will coordinate this effort?

- What is the cost of purchased material versus development of your own?

- How will materials be made readily available for staff?

## REFERENCES

Benefield, L. E. (2002). Evidence-based practice: Basic strategies for success. *Home Healthcare Nurse,* 20(12), 803–807.

Centers for Medicare and Medicaid Services, U.S. Department of Health and Human Services. (2002). Outcome-based quality improvement (OBQI) implementation manual. Baltimore, MD: author.

Fonteyn, M. (2002). Print and online versions of evidence-based nursing: Innovative teaching tools for nurse educators. *Evidence-Based Nursing,* 5(1), 6. Retrieved June 27, 2003 from Infotrac database.

Gingerich, B. S. & Ondeck, D. A. (2000). *Clinical pathways for the multidisciplinary home care team.* Gaithersburg, MD: Aspen.

Goode, C. J., Tanaha, D. J., Krugman, M., O'Connor, P. A., Bailey, C., Deutchman, M. et al. (2000). Outcomes from the use of an evidence-based practice guideline. *Nursing Economics,* 18(4), 202. Retrieved January 8, 2003 from Infotrac database.

Grol, R. & Grimshaw, J. (2003). From best evidence to best practice: Effective implementation of change in patients" care. *The Lancet,* 362(9391), 1228.

Humphrey, C. J. & Malone-Nuzzo, P. (1996). *Orientation to home care nursing.* Gaithersburg, MD: Aspen.

*Merriam-Webster's Collegiate Dictionary (10th ed.).* (2002). Springfield, MA: Merriam-Webster.

National Arthritis Foundation. (2003). Research update archives. Retrieved August 21, 2003 from http://www.arthritis.org/research/research_update/archives.asp.

National Institute on Aging. (2003). About the NIA: History and mission. Retrieved August 21, 2003 from http://www.nia.nih.gov/about/history.htm.

Powell, S. K. (2001). *Advanced case management: Outcomes and beyond.* Philadelphia: Lippincott.

Rice, R. (1998). Key concepts of self-care in the home: Implications for home care nurses. *Geriatric Nursing,* 19(1), 52–54.

Shears, K. H. (2003, Fall). How are best practices identified and adopted? *Network,* 23(1), 7. Retrieved December 15, 2003 from Infotrac database.

Stetler, C. (2001). Updating the Stetler model of research utilization to facilitate evidence-based practice. *Nursing Outlook,* 49(6), 272–278. Retrieved August 22, 2003 from Medline database.

Stevens, K. (2002). Star model of evidence-based practice: Cycle of knowledge transformation. Academic Center for Evidence-Based Nursing. Retrieved August 22, 2003 from http://www.acestar.uthscsa.edu/Goals/model1325.html.

Tinetti, M. E., Baker, D., Gallo, W. T., Nanda, A., Charpentier, P., & O'Leary, J. (2002). Evaluation of restorative care versus usual care for older adults receiving an acute episode of home care. *JAMA,* 287(16), 2098. Retrieved June 27, 2003 from Infotrac database.

U.S. Department of Health and Human Services. (1995). Using clinical practice guidelines to evaluate quality of care (AHCPR Publication no. 95-0045). Rockville, MD: author.

U.S. Department of Health and Human Services. (2000). Clinical practice guideline: Pressure ulcers in adults. Agency for Healthcare Research and Quality. Retrieved August 21, 2003 from http://hstat.nlm.nih.gov/hq/Hquest/db/local.ahcpr.quick.putq/screen.

U.S. Department of Health and Human Services. (2003). AHRQ profile. Retrieved August 25, 2003 from http://www.ahrq.gov/about/profile.htm.

U.S. Department of Health and Human Services. Systems to rate the strength of scientific evidence. (2003). Agency for Healthcare Research and Quality. Retrieved August 26, 2003 from http://www.ahrq.gov/clinic/epcssums/strengthsum/htm.

# CHAPTER 1E

# The Foundation of Outcome-Based Home Care: Outcomes Measurement and Standards of Care

# Critical Link between Outcomes Achieved and the Implementation of Standards of Care

> **CORE TERMS AND CONCEPTS**
>
> - Standards of Care
> - Revision of Standards of Care
> - Outcomes Achieved

## LEARNING OBJECTIVES

Upon completion of this topic, you will be able to:

1. Describe the critical link between clinical outcomes achieved and the implementation of standards of care.
2. Revise agency standards of care as needed according to clinical outcomes achieved.

## AGENCY-SPECIFIC DATA/RESOURCES NEEDED

N/A

Outcomes are written and measured to achieve improvement in quality of care. Standards of care and best practice recommendations are implemented with the intent of achieving better patient outcomes. They go hand-in-hand. When specific standards of care form the basis of the patient's plan of care and are implemented accordingly, corresponding outcomes can be more readily evaluated. It becomes easier to pinpoint areas for performance improvement that need review, investigation, and revision.

If the desired outcome is achieved, then reinforcement of the standards becomes the focus. If the desired outcome is not achieved, a review of the standards and standards implementation becomes the focus of the investigation as to why. Standards of care provision are continually reviewed and revised as appropriate to achieve better outcomes.

Other variables, such as patient environment, mental status, age, progression of disease, compliance/noncompliance, and variance also affect outcomes of care. Investigating also includes reviewing the characteristics of the patient population to which the standards have been applied. These patient characteristics give perspective to your findings. Let's look how this critical link is recognized by an agency that develops a specific standard of care with the intention of improving a particular outcome.

For example, an agency has an increased number of falls with injury in patients 75 years and older in the last 12 months as noted through incident reporting. This outcome is not acceptable to agency managers. Safety checklists are completed routinely for every Medicare patient on admission. Usual instruction (usual care) regarding home safety is provided by the safety checklist. The agency has no formal fall prevention program.

Because of this outcome, agency managers investigate the incident reports thoroughly, trying to establish commonalities of age, gender, time of each incident, and how, why, and where the patient was when the fall occurred. Patient records are also accessed to determine if OASIS responses among this group have any similarities, such as functional impairments on admission, debilitating conditions, orthopedic or musculo-skeletal diagnoses that could affect balance or gait, the use of special equipment, and home environment.

After an investigation of each incident, the agency decides to implement a standard of care to help reduce injury and falls in this patient group. The person responsible for coordinating performance improvement efforts uses the Internet to access the National Guideline Clearinghouse (www.guideline.gov), searching for evidence-based best practices related to fall prevention.

The *Guideline for the Prevention of Falls in Older Persons* of the American Academy of Orthopedic Surgeons (AAOS) in conjunction with the American Geriatric Society (AGS) and the British Geriatrics Society (BGS) includes multifaceted interventions, guidance regarding long-term exercise, and balance training (American Geriatric Society, British Geriatrics Society, and American Academy of Orthopedic Surgeons, 2001). This guideline also directs the PI coordinator to the patient teaching guide entitled, *A Patient's Guide to Preventing Falls*, made available through the AGS (AGS, 2001).

From these resources, several interventions, including fall risk assessment, are found. These improve outcomes by reducing fall and injury in older persons. Several items are brought to the agency's Fall Prevention PI focus group for discussion and evaluation. The group considers several items to include in a standard of care:

- They agree that a fall risk assessment tool is needed and that information from the Clearinghouse Guidelines will be used to develop this tool.
- They agree that clinicians will conduct a fall prevention follow-up each visit for those patients identified at risk. This includes observing for an unsafe environment from the initial assessment and observing to see if recommended changes were made by the patient or caretaker to enhance safety in the home.
- They thoroughly evaluate the AGS teaching material, *A Patient's Guide to Preventing Falls*, and decide to adopt this as the source that will be used by clinicians for patient/caretaker education.

- For those patients at risk for falls, as identified by the risk assessment tool, a physical therapy evaluation will be considered.
- OASIS patient responses will also be reviewed in making this determination. Communication will be documented in the medical record. If the therapist deems that an evaluation is indicated, the physician is contacted. If the physician orders treatment, the therapist uses the information from the guidelines to develop the patient's home program for exercise, strength, and balance, as appropriate.
- They interview staff and conduct chart review to determine the current use of the agency's home safety checklist.
  1. Has the use of this checklist become mundane and lost its importance? Is it simply another form to complete?
  2. Is it out of date and in need of revision?
  3. Does it include recommendations for preventing falls as found in the Guidelines Clearinghouse?
  4. Is it specific for identifying environmental causes of falls?

The PI focus group writes the following agency standards of care for fall prevention in persons 75 years and older:

- All patients 75 years and older are assessed for fall risk on admission, using the agency's fall risk assessment tool.
- All patients identified at risk for falls receive the booklet entitled, *A Patient's Guide to Preventing Falls*, no later than the second visit.
- All patients deemed at risk for falls, as identified by the risk assessment tool and who have OASIS responses indicative of possible risk, are considered for a physical therapy evaluation. Communication is documented in the medical record.

The group discusses ways of incorporating this standard into routine care provision:

- Fall risk assessment is included as part of the admission assessment; it is not to be an additional form.
- OASIS item responses are evaluated for inclusion in the *fall risk assessment* portion of the admission assessment.
- Patients identified at risk for falls are placed on a patient listing and distributed to staff. Listing is updated bi-weekly to include new admissions.
- All patients at risk for falls receiving Home Health Aide (HHA) services will have this notation made on the HHA assignment sheet.
- Clinical visit note includes a brief section for fall prevention. It is completed each visit for those identified for fall risk.

They design an action plan and present the timeline to the agency director. They discuss the plan with the agency's medical director/advisor. The plan includes the following elements:

- Development of the fall risk assessment items.
- Evaluation of clinical forms for location of fall risk assessment and visit notations.
- Adoption of the *A Patient's Guide to Preventing Falls* for use in patient teaching.
- Education of staff regarding the standard of care for fall risk and prevention.
- Education of all clinicians and HHAs regarding their role in the prevention of falls.
- Development and dissemination of fall risk patient listing.
- Quarterly follow-up for the agency outcome, *Falls with Injury*.

The number of falls in this patient group declined substantially over the six months following implementation of the agency's new standard of care. The agency achieved an improvement in this outcome primarily due to the development and implementation of a standard of care to address it. *This demonstrates the critical link.*

After a year of implementation, the agency's outcome for falls with injury in patients 75 years and older begins to rise. The outcome is less than desired; a review of the standard and implementation by staff is once again in order.

*Guiding Questions*

- Have the characteristics of the agency's 75 years and older population changed over the course of the year? Does the patient age that is used need to include those 65 years and older?
- Do incident reports describe a change in the time or location of falls? Contributing factors to falls?
- Are staff applying the standards for every appropriate patient?
- Are staff implementing the standard of care properly?
- Are there new staff that have not been oriented to the use of standard?
- Are staff held accountable for implementing the standard?
- Are staff documenting interventions that are recommended by the standard?
- Are staff experiencing new obstacles or inefficiencies in carrying out the standard?
- Are new staff measuring the outcomes (results) accurately?
- Is the implementation of the standard on evenings and weekends part of the problem?

---

### CONCEPT APPLICATION:
### Linking Standards of Care to Outcomes Achieved

The agency's outcome, *Fall with Injury*, has worsened over the last 12 months for the agency as determined through evaluation of agency incident or unusual occurrence reports and the agency's OBQM Adverse Event Report. Let's discuss two different scenarios that suggest possible causes.

*Scenario 1*

The agency implemented a standard of care for fall prevention one and a half years ago.

1. Through chart review and staff interview you determine that the standard of care is not always implemented properly. You discover that:

   a) Two newly hired nurses do not always initiate the standard of care upon patient admission.
   b) Fall prevention teaching materials are on back order and are frequently unavailable for staff use.
   c) The risk assessment portion of the admission assessment does not receive proper clinician follow-up in three of every five patients admitted.
   d) Patients admitted on weekends do not always have the standard of care initiated.

2. There has been no formal follow-up education for staff since implementing the standard 12 months ago.

3. There has been only a brief mention of occurrence of patient falls in one staff meeting during this past year, according to staff meeting minutes. Awareness of fall prevention has waned.

## CONCEPT APPLICATION:

### Linking Standards of Care to Outcomes Achieved

*(continued)*

In this example, areas needing follow-up include:

- Newly hired nurses initiating the standard upon admission
- Availability of teaching materials
- Breakdown in the process on weekends
- Staff accountability in use of risk assessment tool
- Need to schedule fall risk and prevention education for staff
- Need for discussion of outcome findings in staff meetings and increased awareness.

### Scenario 2

Upon review of the implementation of the standards of care by the staff, you determine that they *are implementing the standards properly*. Then why is there an increase in falls?

To determine why, you review the characteristics of the patient population and find that the majority of these patients are over 75 years old, live alone, have a low frequency of caretaker assistance, and have urinary incontinence at night. Two-thirds of the falls occurred at night while the patient was going to the bathroom. This gives perspective to the outcome achieved and your investigation. This population has changed and may be at a higher risk.

### Guiding Questions

- Do we have a standard of care for urinary incontinence?
- If so, are staff properly implementing this standard of care?
- If not, do we need to obtain or develop a standard of care for incontinence?
- Do revisions in the standard for fall prevention need to include interventions for incontinence management at night?
- Are staff taking proactive steps to evaluate the low frequency of assistance and its effect on the patient's care and recovery?
- Does this group have social service issues in common that require MSS assistance for resolution?

Revise the standard or implementation of the standard accordingly. Monitor the outcome at least quarterly. Locate best practices and develop standards of care according to the specific outcome(s) you want to achieve. Examine all possibilities that you believe can positively affect the outcome in question, realizing that variables in patients and in their environments do exist.

Use performance improvement tools and methods, such as cause and effect diagrams, force-field analysis, multi-voting, and brainstorming (Joint Commission on Accreditation of Healthcare Organizations, 2002) and the Plan-Do-Study-Act (Ramsey, Ormsby, and Marsh, 2000) to help determine why the outcome exists and to decide which standards may have the greatest impact on improving the outcome. Don't lose sight of the critical link when performing this task.

**REFERENCES**

American Geriatric Society. (2001). *A patient's guide to preventing falls*. New York, NY: author.

American Geriatric Society, British Geriatrics Society, and the American Academy of Orthopedic Surgeons. (2001). Guideline for the prevention of falls in older persons. *Journal of American Geriatric Society*, 49(5), 664–672.

Joint Commission on Accreditation of Healthcare Organizations. (2002). *Using performance improvement tools in health care settings*. Revised Edition. Oakbrook Terrace, IL: Joint Commission Resources.

Ramsey, C., Ormsby, S., & Marsh, T. (2000, December). Performance improvement strategies can reduce costs. *Healthcare Financial Management*. Retrieved December 23, 2003 from http://www.findarticles.com/cf_dls/m3257/12_54/68215551/p1/article.jhtml.

# CHAPTER 2A

# Building an Outcome-Based Approach to Home Care

# Getting Started: Defining Your Agency's Patient Population(s) and Evaluating Related Staff Experience and Expertise

**CORE TERMS AND CONCEPTS**

- Patient Population
- Top Primary Diagnoses
- Patient Demographics/ Characteristics
- Co-Morbid Conditions

## LEARNING OBJECTIVES

Upon completion of this topic, you will able to:

1. Identify your agency's top diagnoses in the past 12 months according to admission volume.
2. Identify the characteristics that describe your patients with these diagnoses.
3. Evaluate special work experience and expertise of all levels of staff in relation to your agency's patient population(s).
4. Determine if additional diagnoses warrant an allocation of resources for outcome-based patient management.

## AGENCY-SPECIFIC DATA/RESOURCES NEEDED

1. Diagnoses by admission volume in descending order over the past 12 months. (Accessed from the agency's database of information.)
2. Staff special work experience and/or training from surveys or personnel files.

# INTRODUCTION

Successful implementation of an outcome-based approach to home care begins by defining the *primary patient population(s)* ("Joint Commission looking for," 2003) served by the agency. Then the agency can determine where it can have the greatest impact on quality improvement. A small agency may identify one or two primary patient populations or groups, while a large agency may have several. There is no specific number of populations that your agency should strive to identify.

One of the biggest missteps an agency can make is identifying too many patient types, diagnoses, or procedures, or in some cases, not identifying populations at all. When an inordinate number of patient groups is identified, managing data related to these groups becomes too burdensome and may not be of real value to the agency. Not identifying populations at all can result in missed opportunities for performance improvement and in more efficient use of resources. The key is to focus on a *select few* patient groups, especially during the early transition to outcome-based care delivery.

## IDENTIFYING PATIENT POPULATIONS

Primary patient populations can be selected through one or a combination of activities. These include:

- identifying primary diagnoses or conditions by admission volume (Peters, Cowley, and Standiford, 1999; Smith, 2001).
- identifying those diagnoses or conditions that entail problematic or high-risk treatment or procedures.
- identifying those diagnoses, conditions, or procedures that incur high cost ("Select where you can have an impact," 2002).
- reviewing patient demographics and characteristics (Tinetti, Baker, Gallo, Nanda, Charpentier, and O'Leary, 2002).

### Identifying Primary Diagnoses and Conditions by Volume

High volume diagnoses must have ongoing attention (Smith, 2001) as they typically generate the majority of your revenue and often represent *difficult to manage* chronic conditions. Because primary diagnoses in an agency periodically change, you should start by evaluating the past 12 months of agency data. Take note of the top ten ICD-9 primary diagnoses; as you review this list, Arslanian (2001) recommends asking these guiding questions:

- Does the benefit of providing outcome-based care for a particular diagnosis or condition outweigh the cost and effort of providing it?
- Will the data from a particular patient population be meaningful?

### Identifying Diagnoses or Conditions That Entail Problematic or High-Risk Treatment/Procedures

To pinpoint previous problem areas, review past performance improvement (PI) initiatives, adverse events, and patient complaints. Also consider populations whose care requires high-risk interventions such as enteral, parenteral, or vascular infusion therapy, vascular access device insertion and care, complex wound care, and management of communicable diseases. Any new procedures or those in which problems have occurred are always worthy of attention.

# Reviewing Demographics and Other Patient Characteristics

Patient demographics are characteristics or descriptors that describe a patient population (i.e., age, gender, geographical location, and payer source) (Merriam-Webster, 2002). Ethnicity and language may also be used. These demographics change as your community changes, making it necessary to review them periodically (Smith, 2001). Powell (2001) recommends including the factors of age, diagnosis, gender, and co-morbidities when describing patient populations. Co-morbid conditions or co-morbidities, as they are often called, are *those that are secondary, often complicating primary treatment and increasing the risk of other related conditions* (Coon and Zulkowski, 2002). For example, patients with diabetes often have the co-morbidity of heart disease.

Strickland (1997) recommends knowing the characteristics of the population(s) served when planning interventions and when looking at outcomes. For example, if an agency cares for a large number of pediatric patients with failure to thrive who live in an economically depressed area, it is prudent that the agency provide interventions and measure outcomes related to nutrition, hydration, weight, bonding, and developmental stage. While this may seem obvious in this example, consider an all-adult population, where the lines become more blurred.

At first glance it may seem neither practical nor justified to allocate resources for the interventions and measurement of outcomes related to a special return-to-work rehabilitation program for a small number of patients, especially when 72% of your patients are 75 years of age or older and are retired. However, if offering a return-to-work program addresses a need for a small community work force, where a single industry provides most of the income for young families, then this patient population takes on more significance and may be worthy of agency resources.

Other characteristics or descriptors are often used in addition to demographics when describing patients, as seen in OBQI/OBQM (DHHS, 2002). OASIS responses provide additional characteristics of the patients you serve, e.g., Primary Caregiver, Current Living Situation, Therapies received at Home, and Chronic Conditions (CMS, 2002). These are provided in the OBQI report: *Case Mix Profile.*

For example, administering infusion therapy to a moderate number of adult patients who have no single primary caretaker may substantiate the need for greater resources and attention to processes of care because of the potential risks involved with this intervention given the circumstances.

*Note: The Case Mix Profile report will be discussed in detail in Section B of this chapter.*

**2**A

## AGENCY APPLICATION:
### Identifying Agency Primary Patient Populations

Identify your primary patient population(s) by first listing the agency's top ten ICD-9 primary diagnoses over the last 12 months in descending order according to admission volume. Beside each diagnosis enter the number of patient admissions and the percentage of admissions by diagnosis relative to total admissions for the same time period.

| Diagnosis | No. of Admissions | % of Total Admissions |
|---|---|---|
| 1. | | |
| 2. | | |
| 3. | | |
| 4. | | |
| 5. | | |
| 6. | | |
| 7. | | |
| 8. | | |
| 9. | | |
| 10. | | |

*Guiding Questions*

- What characteristics do the majority of your patients who have each of these diagnoses share: What is the average age? What is the gender? Where do the patients live?
- Do the majority live alone? Assisted living?
- Is there use of a secondary language? What are the cultures represented?
- What resources do you have to manage patients of different cultures in our service area(s)?
- What are your primary referral sources relative to your top diagnoses? Hospital discharge planners, case managers, physicians, other practitioners? Do some physicians travel from out-of-town to see patients in a weekly clinic setting?
- Are there other diagnoses for which you want to provide outcome-based care? What is your rationale? Is it to control costs? To address a quality issue? To prepare for a new group of incoming physicians? To build a hospital-home health joint continuum of care for a particular patient population, such as pediatric asthma, CHF, COPD, diabetes, joint replacement?

## AGENCY APPLICATION:
### Identifying Agency Primary Patient Populations *(continued)*

Finally, consider the patient populations that you plan to serve in the future. These may be targeted through business development efforts, new hospital services offered in the community, needs expressed by physician customers, discharge planners, and other consumers of the agency's services. Add additional diagnoses or substitute a diagnosis in the place of another if rationale supports this. As your agency becomes more sophisticated in defining its populations, others may be added as needed.

## EVALUATING STAFF EXPERIENCE AND EXPERTISE

Once you have defined your patient population(s), re-evaluate special talents and expertise of your clinical staff in relation to these patient populations served. These staff members can be an important clinical resource in the transition to outcome-based patient care. Hidden talent is often buried within a resume or application.

For example, an agency has a high volume of patients with diagnoses related to wounds, incontinence, and respiratory illness. It currently provides usual care to these patients. The agency does not have access to a wound-ostomy-continence specialty nurse. A review of staff work history and survey reveals that one RN previously worked in an outpatient respiratory clinic and that an LPN was on the wound care team of the local hospital.

The agency has identified two individuals with expertise beyond the provision of usual care. These staff members can provide valuable suggestions to managers regarding the care of the patients who are driving a large portion of the revenue. Have them assist in evaluating the care that is currently being provided to the wound patients and to those with respiratory illness. Involve them in developing the standards of care for these high volume diagnoses and in performance improvement initiatives designed to improve or maintain desired outcomes. The agency may also have staff that wishes to provide direct patient care to these particular types of patients, given the opportunity. They can act as potential preceptors to orient new staff, as well as assist with education and competency.

**2**A

## AGENCY APPLICATION:

### Evaluating Related Work Experience and Expertise

Evaluate your staff clinical work experience and special skills related to your agency's primary populations. Review applications and resumes or conduct a quick and simple survey. List the employee's name, title, and his or her special skills.

For example:

Jane Doe, RN       *Cardiac rehabilitation—urban medical center—one year*
John Doe, COTA     *Inpatient rehab; worked with hip/knee replacements*

Name & Title        Special Skills/Experience

1. _____

2. _____

3. _____

4. _____

5. _____

6. _____

7. _____

### Guiding Questions

- Are staff experience and expertise being used to the fullest potential allowed by your state practice act, relative to providing the care required by your primary populations?
- Are staff experience and expertise used to enhance the provision of care through involvement in performance improvement?

**REFERENCES**

Arslanian, C. (2001). Developing an orthopaedic outcomes program. *Orthopaedic Nursing,* 20(92), 19. Retrieved January 8, 2003 from Infotrac database.

Centers for Medicare and Medicaid Services, U.S. Department of Health and Human Services. (Dec. 2002). Outcome-based quality improvement (OBQI) implementation manual. Baltimore, MD: author.

Coon, P. & Zulkowski, K. (2002). Adherence to American Diabetes Association standards of care by rural health providers. *Diabetes Care,* 25(12), 2224. Retrieved August 15, 2003 from Infotrac database.

Joint Commission looking for outcomes measurement: Should be a high priority for patient educators. (2003). *Patient Education Management,* 10(1), 4.

*Merriam-Webster's Collegiate Dictionary (10th ed.).* (2002). Merriam-Webster, Inc.

Peters, C., Cowley, M., & Standiford, L. (1999). The process of outcomes management in an acute care facility. *Nursing Administration Quarterly,* 24(1), 75. Retrieved April 16, 2003 from Infotrac database.

Powell, S. K. (2001). *Advanced case management: Outcomes and beyond.* Philadelphia: Lippincott.

Select where you can have impact on cost & utilization: Develop your DM program one step at a time. (2002). *Case Management Advisor,* 13(5), 51. Retrieved April 16, 2003 from Infotrac database.

Smith, A. P. (2001). Removing the fluff: The quality in quality improvement. *Nursing Economics,* 19(4), 183. Retrieved April 14, 2003 from Infotrac database.

Strickland, O. L. (1997). Challenges in measuring patient outcomes. In S. Prevost (Ed.), *The Nursing Clinics of North America: Outcomes measurement and management.* (pp. 495–512). Philadelphia: W. B. Saunders.

Tinetti, M. E., Baker, D., Gallo, W. T., Nanda, A., Charpentier, P., & O'Leary, J. (2002). Evaluation of restorative care versus usual care for older adults receiving an acute episode of home care. *JAMA,* 287(16), 2098. Retrieved April 14, 2003 from Infotrac database.

# CHAPTER 2B

# Building an Outcome-Based Approach to Home Care

# OASIS Outcomes and Outcome-Based Quality Improvement (OBQI)

## LEARNING OBJECTIVES

Upon completion of this topic, you will be able to:

1. Differentiate OBQI from OBQM.
2. Analyze and interpret:
   • a Case Mix Profile Report
   • a Risk-Adjusted and Descriptive Outcome Report
   • an Adverse Event Outcome Report
3. Select an OASIS OBQI target outcome for investigation.
4. Prioritize OBQM adverse events outcomes for investigation.
5. Select patients from Tally Reports for record review.
6. Select queries for the Tally Report Workbook tool.
7. Conduct an OASIS outcomes investigation.
8. Integrate OASIS outcome findings into clinical practice.

---

**CORE TERMS AND CONCEPTS**

- OBQI/OBQM
- Case Mix Profile Report
- Adverse Event Outcome Report
- Adverse Event—Patient Listing
- Risk-Adjusted and Descriptive Outcome Report
- Patient Tally Report
- Tally Report Workbook Tool
- Target Outcome
- Outcome (Process of Care) Investigation

---

## AGENCY-SPECIFIC DATA/RESOURCES NEEDED

1. Your agency's OBQI Case Mix Profile Report and Case Mix Tally Report for the last 12 months.
2. OBQI Risk-Adjusted and Descriptive Outcome Report and Outcome Tally Report for the same period.
3. OBQI Adverse Event Outcome Report and Adverse Event Patient Listing for the same period.

# INTRODUCTION

The information here is presented in a quick reference format so that you can readily access the steps and activities of OBQI/OBQM used in the remaining examples of this workbook. It also provides the nuts and bolts of how to read OBQI/OBQM reports, how to select OASIS outcomes for performance improvement, how to select patient medical records for chart review, and how to investigate OASIS outcomes data.

The outcomes measured through OASIS and improved or reinforced through OBQI can also be integrated into other outcome-based methods, such as care pathways and disease management (DM). These are discussed in Sections C and D of this chapter.

*Note: It is beyond the scope and purpose of this text to provide an all-inclusive discussion of OBQI and OBQM. For comprehensive detail, refer to the CMS OBQI Implementation Manual and its Supplements. The manual and supplements can be downloaded from the following website: http://www.cms.hhs.gov/oasis/obqi.asp.*

## OASIS OUTCOMES AND OBQI/OBQM OUTCOME REPORTS

The use of OASIS was mandated by CMS to enable rigorous and systematic measurement of home health patient outcomes, with appropriate adjustment for patient risk factors affecting those outcomes (CMS, 2002). Outcomes have become the ultimate *yardstick* by which home care quality is measured and agencies are compared.

OASIS outcomes are the basis of OBQI and OBQM. Both are systematic approaches that agencies can implement to continuously improve the quality of care they provide ( CMS, 2002). OBQI seeks to use Risk-Adjusted Outcomes to indicate whether a patient's condition has improved or stabilized over time, such as *Improvement in bathing, Improvement in dyspnea,* and *Stabilization in transferring.* For example, a patient who required assistance to bathe in the shower or tub at the start of care (SOC) and who is now able to bathe self has achieved the outcome of *Improvement in bathing.*

OBQM entails more direct measurements of the occurrence of adverse events. Adverse Event Outcomes serve as red flags for potential problems of a negative nature and occur in relatively low frequency (e.g., *Increase in the number of pressure ulcers, Development of urinary tract infection,* and *Emergent care for injury caused by fall or accident at home).* Adverse event outcomes are used to monitor the progress an agency makes in addressing negative occurrences. For example, an agency has a disturbingly high percentage of patients requiring *Emergent care for hypo/hyperglycemia.* The agency addresses this issue through PI and monitors this outcome periodically to determine if it is improving.

OASIS outcome measurements are obtained and calculated directly from the patient/family/caretaker responses to OASIS data set items. The calculation is made from any change that has occurred in the patient's health status between two or more OASIS response time points (i.e., SOC, resumption of care, other follow-up, transfer, and discharge). Outcome measurements are potentially affected by the patient's consistent or changing responses.

These responses are combined as a whole *(aggregated)* into outcomes through OASIS software and provided to each agency as outcome reports. For example, responses to OASIS item *MO490: When is the patient dyspneic or noticeably short of breath?* are aggregated by OASIS software as the basis for the end-result outcome of *Improvement in dyspnea.*

These reports are used to compare an agency's outcomes to those reported in the prior year and to a national reference mean (CMS, 2002). These reports are available for use by agency managers to:

- pinpoint areas of patient care that need improvement
- reinforce maintenance of positive outcomes achieved
- investigate problematic areas
- allocate resources more appropriately

- enhance staff development offerings
- evaluate staff competency

Accurately analyzing and interpreting the OBQI/OBQM reports is essential to integrating OASIS outcomes into clinical practice. The OBQI/OBQM reports include:

- Case Mix Profile Report (used in OBQI & OBQM)
- Risk-Adjusted and Descriptive Outcome Report (used for OBQI)
- Patient Tally Reports
- Adverse Event Outcome Report (used for OBQM)
- Adverse Event Patient Listing

## Case Mix Profile Report

This report aggregates the demographics, characteristics, conditions, disabilities, and diseases of patients admitted to an agency within a specific time period (CMS, 2002). It provides a general description of the Medicare/Medicaid patient population served. Because this report describes the patient population, and gives perspective to the outcomes, it should be used in conjunction with other OBQI/OBQM reports. This information may also be used for resource allocation and changing staff mix, modifying policy or procedures, and determining the need for care pathway development and strategic planning (Health Care Financing Administration [HCFA], 2001).

For example, a Case Mix Profile Report reveals that an agency has a large number of elderly patients with incontinence. This information prompts the agency to pay particular attention to the OASIS outcomes that are functional and physiologic in nature, i.e., *Improvement in toileting* and *Improvement in urinary incontinence*. This finding also causes the agency to take a closer look at the skilled care provided for incontinent patients and home health aide services and training related to incontinent care. *Note: Make sure that the Case Mix Profile Report is run for the same time period as the other outcome reports you are reviewing.*

### Report Format and Description

See Figure 2.1 on the following page for format of Case Mix Profile Report. The item numbers used below correspond to the circled numbers you see in Figure 2.1. For this discussion, also refer to **your agency's** Case Mix Profile Report for the past 12 months.

The Case Mix Profile has two columns that give patient characteristics for the last 12 months, such as demographics, payment source, ADL status prior to SOC/ROC, and current residence.

1. To the immediate right of each characteristic is its **current mean expressed as a percentage or as a decimal**.
   a. The **current average** being reported for patients is expressed as a percent. For example, in Figure 2.1, 13.98% of these patients reported had intractable pain.
   b. The **current average scale score** of an attribute for patients being reported is expressed as a decimal. For example, in Figure 2.1, a patient's ability to transfer is described on a scale of 0–5 for OASIS *(M0690)* as 0.64. In general, the higher the average scale score or decimal number, the more impairment exists for the patients being reported.
2. To the right of the agency's current mean is the **Prior Mean** or agency's case mix average from the prior 12-month period.
3. To the right of the agency's prior mean is the **Reference (Ref.) mean**. The reference mean is the average of the national sample of all patients from all agencies submitting data.
   *Note: All means are expressed as a percent or decimal.*

## Figure 2.1  Case Mix Profile Report

**Agency Name:** FAIRCARE HOME HEALTH SERVICES
**Agency ID:** HHA01
**Location:** ANYTOWN, USA
**Medicare Number:** 007001
**Medicaid Number:** 999888001
**Date Report Printed:** 03/21/2003

**Requested Current Period:** 01/2002 - 12/2002
**Requested Prior Period:** 01/2001 - 12/2001
**Actual Current Period:** 01/2002 - 12/2002
**Actual Prior Period:** 01/2001 - 12/2001
**# Cases:** Curr 601   Prior 551
**Number of Cases in Reference Segment:** 3289067

### Case Mix Profile at Start/Resumption of Care
For Risk-Adjusted/Descriptive Outcome Report

| | Current Mean | Prior Mean | Ref. Mean | | Current Mean | Prior Mean | Ref. Mean |
|---|---|---|---|---|---|---|---|
| **Demographics** | | | | **ADL Status Prior to SOC/ROC** | | | |
| Age (average in years) | 70.75 | 70.98 | 72.78 * | Grooming (0-3, scale average) | 0.56 | 0.68 | 0.52 * |
| Gender: Female (%) | 69.38% | 66.62% | 62.89% ** | Dress upper body (0-3, scale avg.) | 0.35 | 0.32 | 0.35 |
| Race: Black (%) | 1.66% | 1.63% | 10.71% ** | Dress lower body (0-3, scale avg.) | 0.70 | 0.76 + | 0.63 |
| Race: White (%) | 97.50% | 97.84% | 85.48% ** | Bathing (0-5, scale avg.) | 1.33 | 1.26 | 1.20 |
| Race: Other (%) | 0.83% | 0.67% | 3.82% ** | Toileting (0-4, scale avg.) | 0.39 | 0.40 | 0.38 |
| | | | | Transferring (0-5, scale avg.) | 0.38 | 0.37 | 0.44 * |
| **Payment Source** | | | | Ambulation (0-5, scale avg.) | 0.70 | 0.72 | 0.71 * |
| Any Medicare (%) | 80.43% | 81.48% | 82.59% | Eating (0-5, scale avg.) | 0.22 | 0.22 | 0.21 |
| Any Medicaid (%) | 12.88% | 14.44% | 14.30% | | | | |
| Any HMO (%) | 3.01% | 2.87% | 5.76% ** | **IADL Disabilities at SOC/ROC** | | | |
| Medicare HMO (%) | 1.34% | 1.15% | 2.23% | Light meal prep (0-2, scale avg.) | 1.02 | 1.02 | 0.90 |
| Any third party (%) | 19.90% | 23.47% | 21.90% | Transportation (0-2, scale avg.) | 1.05 | 1.04 | 0.99 |
| | | | | Laundry (0-2, scale avg.) | 1.62 | 1.49 | 1.51 |
| **Current Residence** | | | | Housekeeping (0-4, scale avg.) | 2.89 | 2.68 | 2.68 |
| Own home (%) | 74.70% | 73.07% | 78.65% * | Shopping (0-3, scale avg.) | 2.10 | 1.90 | 2.06 * |
| Family member home (%) | 20.53% | 21.05% | 14.11% ** | Phone (0-5, scale avg.) | 0.63 | 0.60 | 0.72 * |
| | | | | Mgmt. oral meds (0-2, scale avg.) | 0.69 | 0.69 | 0.70 |
| **Current Living Situation** | | | | | | | |
| Lives alone (%) | 28.62% | 31.17% | 29.42% | **IADL Status Prior to SOC/ROC** | | | |
| With family member (%) | 66.72% | 62.77% | 64.23% | Light meal prep (0-2, scale avg.) | 0.65 | 0.60 | 0.56 |
| With friend (%) | 1.33% | 1.27% | 1.62% | Transportation (0-2, scale avg.) | 0.78 | 0.82 | 0.69 |
| With paid help (%) | 2.33% | 2.03% | 3.28% | Laundry (0-2, scale avg.) | 1.10 | 1.01 | 0.96 |
| | | | | Housekeeping (0-4, scale avg.) | 1.93 | 1.77 | 1.73 |
| **Assisting Persons** | | | | Shopping (0-3, scale avg.) | 1.45 | 1.42 | 1.32 |
| Person residing in home (%) | 57.00% | 62.12% | 55.94% | Phone (0-5, scale avg.) | 0.49 | 0.51 | 0.59 * |
| Person residing outside home (%) | 44.33% | 50.52% + | 53.00% ** | Mgmt. oral meds (0-2, scale avg.) | 0.53 | 0.55 | 0.54 |
| Paid help (%) | 9.33% | 9.59% | 14.09% ** | | | | |
| | | | | **Respiratory Status** | | | |
| **Primary Caregiver** | | | | Dyspnea (0-4, scale avg.) | 1.33 | 1.26 | 1.19 * |
| Spouse/significant other (%) | 31.00% | 30.42% | 33.58% | | | | |
| Daughter/son (%) | 33.00% | 28.01% | 26.37% ** | **Therapies Received at Home** | | | |
| Other paid help (%) | 3.67% | 2.78% | 6.05% * | IV/infusion therapy (%) | 4.33% | 4.24% | 3.74% |
| No one person (%) | 21.67% | 21.76% | 20.19% | Parenteral nutrition (%) | 0.50% | 0.50% | 0.28% |
| | | | | Enteral nutrition (%) | 2.16% | 2.18% | 1.75% |
| **Primary Caregiver Assistance** | | | | | | | |
| Freq. of assistance (0-6, scale avg.) | 4.11 | 4.05 | 4.10 | **Sensory Status** | | | |
| | | | | Vision impairment (0-2, scale avg.) | 0.32 | 0.34 | 0.30 |
| **Inpatient DC within 14 Days of SOC/ROC** | | | | Hearing impair. (0-4, scale avg.) | 0.38 | 0.39 | 0.45 * |
| From hospital (%) | 69.05% | 66.56% | 68.41% | Speech/language (0-5, scale avg.) | 0.45 | 0.48 | 0.47 |
| From rehab facility (%) | 7.15% | 6.99% | 6.38% | | | | |
| From nursing home (%) | 1.83% | 1.59% | 3.28% | **Pain** | | | |
| | | | | Pain interf. w/activity (0-3, scale avg.) | 0.95 | 0.98 | 0.98 |
| **Med. Reg. Chg. w/in 14 Days of SOC/ROC** | | | | Intractable pain (%) | 13.98% | 13.28% | 13.69% |
| Medical regimen change (%) | 67.72% | 74.56% + | 81.21% ** | | | | |
| | | | | **Neuro/Emotional/Behavioral Status** | | | |
| **Prognoses** | | | | Moderate cognitive disability (%) | 10.82% | 7.82% | 11.91% |
| Moderate recovery prognosis (%) | 85.26% | 82.19% | 85.87% | Severe confusion disability (%) | 5.66% | 7.67% | 6.87% |
| Good rehab prognosis (%) | 62.63% | 64.06% | 68.24% ** | Severe anxiety level (%) | 16.69% | 20.48% | 11.68% * |
| | | | | Behav probs > twice a week (%) | 13.98% | 12.36% | 5.56% * |
| **ADL Disabilities at SOC/ROC** | | | | | | | |
| Grooming (0-3, scale average) | 1.02 | 1.07 | 0.66 * | **Integumentary Status** | | | |
| Dress upper body (0-3, scale avg.) | 0.56 | 0.50 | 0.59 | Presence of wound/lesion (%) | 31.61% | 33.95% | 31.20% |
| Dress lower body (0-3, scale avg.) | 1.22 | 1.19 | 1.10 | Stasis ulcer(s) present (%) | 3.66% | 4.33% | 2.88% |
| Bathing (0-5, scale avg.) | 2.15 | 2.34 | 2.03 | Surgical wounds(s) present (%) | 21.13% | 18.74% | 22.33% |
| Toileting (0-4, scale avg.) | 0.63 | 0.59 | 0.57 | Pressure ulcer(s) present (%) | 8.15% | 7.09% | 5.35% * |
| Transferring (0-5, scale avg.) | 0.64 | 0.63 | 0.70 * | Stage 2-4 ulcer(s) present (%) | 6.49% | 7.98% | 4.54% * |
| Ambulation (0-5, scale avg.) | 1.05 | 1.13 | 1.07 | Stage 3-4 ulcer(s) present (%) | 3.99% | 4.49% | 1.42% * |
| Eating (0-5, scale avg.) | 0.33 | 0.33 | 0.32 | | | | |

4. The **Prior Mean** has a **significance level noted as + or ++**.
One or two *plus signs* displayed here indicate that the probability is greater than or equal to 95% that the difference is **real**, not due to chance.
5. The **Reference Mean** has its **significance level noted by * or ***.
One or two *asterisks* displayed here indicates that the probability of the difference in the agency's average and the reference average is 99%–99.9% **real**, not due to chance. Significance is a statistical comparison between two sets of patient cases that is converted to a percentage.

---

### AGENCY APPLICATION:
### Reading the Case Mix Profile Report

1. Review all patient characteristics in your agency's Case Mix Profile Report for the last 12 months.
2. Highlight those characteristics that have asterisks (* or **) that indicate significance is likely real.
3. Compare each highlighted characteristic to its corresponding national reference mean.

*Guiding Questions*

- How is your population similar to the national sample of patients?
- How is it different?
- After reviewing your agency's Case Mix Profile Report, how would you describe your agency's patient population for this report period?
- Do any of the characteristics of your agency's patient population surprise you?

---

**2**B

## Risk-Adjusted and Descriptive Outcome Report for OBQI

This report is divided into two sections that are downloaded separately—the Risk-Adjusted outcomes, followed by the Descriptive outcomes. The Descriptive outcomes will be *risk-adjusted* in the future and appear separately in the second part of this report (Crisler and Richard, 2002b). Before we continue to describe this report in detail, let's discuss risk adjustment.

Risk adjustment is *a statistical approach that considers the patient characteristics and risk factors most closely associated with specific outcome measures* (Crisler and Richard, 2002b). Risk adjustment controls potential influences that case mix (risk factors) can have upon outcomes. *It minimizes the possibility that differences in outcomes between comparison groups are due to factors other than the care provided by the agency* (CMS, 2002).

For example, an agency's outcomes are less than desired. The agency believes this is caused in part by its patient population being older and having more debilitating chronic conditions than most. Risk adjustment of this agency's outcomes will factor in these patient characteristics when determining their outcome results. OBQI recognizes that certain patients are more or less likely to experience various kinds of outcomes and provides risk adjustment for an *apples-to-apples* comparison between the agency's outcome percentages and the reference sample. This is performed statistically through OASIS software.

*Report Format and Description*

See Figure 2.2 for the format of the Risk-Adjusted and Descriptive Outcome Report. The item numbers used below correspond to the circled numbers in Figure 2.2.

For this discussion, also refer to **your agency's** Risk-Adjusted and Descriptive Outcome Report for the past 12 months.

1. The **report title**.
2. The **key** to the Bar graph.
3. This outcome report has **two categories of outcome measures** listed in a column to the far left side of the page. **End-result** outcomes are reported first, followed by **Utilization** outcomes.
   - **End-result** outcomes relate to the patient's health status, such as functional, cognitive, physiological, and emotional (CMS, 2002). There are two types of end-result outcomes: *improvement* outcomes and *stabilization* outcomes.
      a. A patient ***improves*** in an outcome measure when his or her condition improves between two compared time points (Crisler and Richard, 2002b). Some of these outcome measures are *Improvement in Bathing, Improvement in Eating*, and *Improvement in Bowel Incontinence*.
      b. A patient ***stabilizes*** in an outcome measure when the patient has not worsened between two time points. Some of these outcome measures are *Stabilization in grooming, Stabilization in bathing*, and *Stabilization in transferring*.
   - **Utilization outcomes** relate to the use of healthcare services resulting from a change in patient health status (Crisler and Richard, 2002b) and include *Emergent care provided, Acute care hospitalization*, and *Discharge to community*. Utilization outcomes are computed for all patients, as all patients have the potential to receive emergent care, acute care, or be discharged (CMS, 2002).
4. **Bar Graphs**: Shading indicates the percentage of patient cases relative to the outcome in question.
   - The ***first bar***, with no shading, entitled ***Current***, denotes the agency's outcome percentages for the most recent 12 months. In addition to the percentage, the actual number of agency *current cases*, in which the outcome was achieved, is presented in parentheses at the end of the bar (Chrisler and Richard, 2002b).
   - The ***second bar***, with medium shading, entitled ***Adjusted Prior***, denotes the agency's Risk-Adjusted outcome percentages for the prior 12 months. In the Descriptive outcomes section, it simply reads ***Prior***. (Descriptive outcomes have not all been risk-adjusted at the time of this writing). Adjusted Prior and Prior outcomes allow you to trend your progress on a particular outcome over time (Crisler, Baillie, and Conway, 2003).
   - The ***third bar***, with dark shading, represents the agency's expected percentage given specific case mix or risk factors for Risk-Adjusted outcomes and the reference sample average percentage for Descriptive outcomes.
5. Look to the immediate right of the outcome measures or indicators, and you see the column entitled **Elig. Cases (Eligible Cases)**. There are three numbers given for each outcome. The top number reflects the agency's total number of eligible patients for which the outcome percentage is reported. The second number is the agency's eligible cases for the prior 12 months. The bottom number reflects the total number of patient cases in the national reference sample. When selecting *OBQI Target* outcomes for further investigation, choose only those that have a minimum of 30 cases reported, so the possibility of artificially high percentage results due to a small sample size is lessened.

## Figure 2.2  Risk-Adjusted and Descriptive Outcome Report

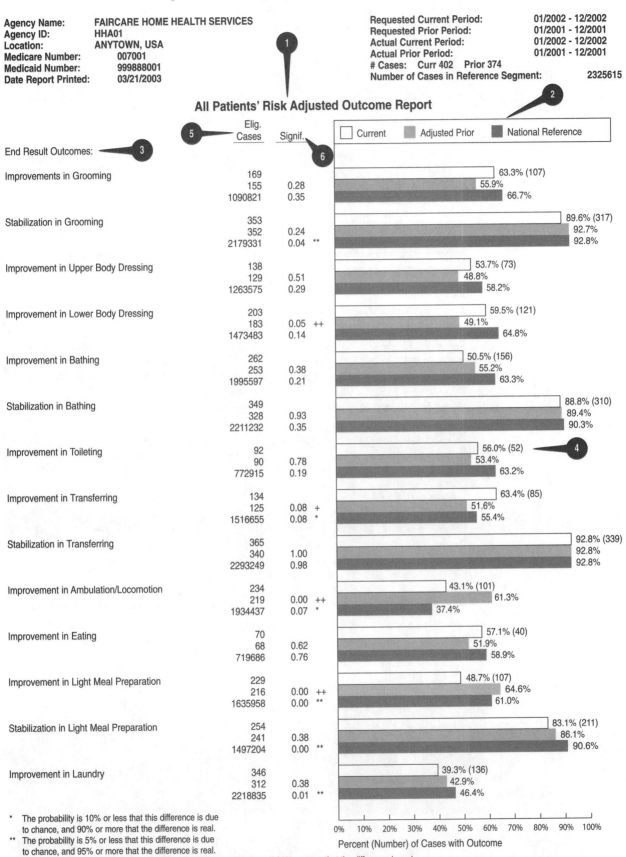

Agency Name:        FAIRCARE HOME HEALTH SERVICES
Agency ID:          HHA01
Location:           ANYTOWN, USA
Medicare Number:    007001
Medicaid Number:    999888001
Date Report Printed: 03/21/2003

Requested Current Period:   01/2002 - 12/2002
Requested Prior Period:     01/2001 - 12/2001
Actual Current Period:      01/2002 - 12/2002
Actual Prior Period:        01/2001 - 12/2001
# Cases:   Curr 402   Prior 374
Number of Cases in Reference Segment:   2325615

### All Patients' Risk Adjusted Outcome Report

Legend: Current | Adjusted Prior | National Reference

| End Result Outcomes: | Elig. Cases | Signif. | Percent (Number) of Cases with Outcome |
|---|---|---|---|
| Improvements in Grooming | 169 | | 63.3% (107) |
| | 155 | 0.28 | 55.9% |
| | 1090821 | 0.35 | 66.7% |
| Stabilization in Grooming | 353 | | 89.6% (317) |
| | 352 | 0.24 | 92.7% |
| | 2179331 | 0.04 ** | 92.8% |
| Improvement in Upper Body Dressing | 138 | | 53.7% (73) |
| | 129 | 0.51 | 48.8% |
| | 1263575 | 0.29 | 58.2% |
| Improvement in Lower Body Dressing | 203 | | 59.5% (121) |
| | 183 | 0.05 ++ | 49.1% |
| | 1473483 | 0.14 | 64.8% |
| Improvement in Bathing | 262 | | 50.5% (156) |
| | 253 | 0.38 | 55.2% |
| | 1995597 | 0.21 | 63.3% |
| Stabilization in Bathing | 349 | | 88.8% (310) |
| | 328 | 0.93 | 89.4% |
| | 2211232 | 0.35 | 90.3% |
| Improvement in Toileting | 92 | | 56.0% (52) |
| | 90 | 0.78 | 53.4% |
| | 772915 | 0.19 | 63.2% |
| Improvement in Transferring | 134 | | 63.4% (85) |
| | 125 | 0.08 + | 51.6% |
| | 1516655 | 0.08 * | 55.4% |
| Stabilization in Transferring | 365 | | 92.8% (339) |
| | 340 | 1.00 | 92.8% |
| | 2293249 | 0.98 | 92.8% |
| Improvement in Ambulation/Locomotion | 234 | | 43.1% (101) |
| | 219 | 0.00 ++ | 61.3% |
| | 1934437 | 0.07 * | 37.4% |
| Improvement in Eating | 70 | | 57.1% (40) |
| | 68 | 0.62 | 51.9% |
| | 719686 | 0.76 | 58.9% |
| Improvement in Light Meal Preparation | 229 | | 48.7% (107) |
| | 216 | 0.00 ++ | 64.6% |
| | 1635958 | 0.00 ** | 61.0% |
| Stabilization in Light Meal Preparation | 254 | | 83.1% (211) |
| | 241 | 0.38 | 86.1% |
| | 1497204 | 0.00 ** | 90.6% |
| Improvement in Laundry | 346 | | 39.3% (136) |
| | 312 | 0.38 | 42.9% |
| | 2218835 | 0.01 ** | 46.4% |

Percent (Number) of Cases with Outcome: 0% 10% 20% 30% 40% 50% 60% 70% 80% 90% 100%

\*   The probability is 10% or less that this difference is due
     to chance, and 90% or more that the difference is real.
\*\*  The probability is 5% or less that this difference is due
     to chance, and 95% or more that the difference is real.
\+   The probability is 10% or less that this difference is due to chance, and 90% or more that the difference is real.
\++  The probability is 5% or less that this difference is due to chance, and 95% or more that the difference is real.

2B

6. The **Signif. (Significance)** of each outcome measure is located to the immediate right of the number of Elig. Cases. A significance of .10 or less indicates a greater probability that the outcome is real and not due to chance.

- For the Current and National Reference comparisons, the significance levels between .05 and .10 are marked with a single *, while those with .05 or less are marked with two **.
- For the *Adjusted Prior* (for Risk-adjusted outcomes) and *Prior* (for Descriptive outcomes), significance levels between .05 and .10 are marked with a single +, while those with .05 or less are marked with ++.
- Identifying significance levels with one * or two ** or with one + or two ++ should always be the first step in selecting *Target* outcomes for evaluation and investigation.
- *Significance levels of .10 or less are those of high priority.* If significance levels are not within this range, then choose those levels closest to .10, but not above .25.

---

## AGENCY APPLICATION:

### Reading the Risk-Adjusted and Descriptive Outcome Report

1. Review your agency's Risk-Adjusted and Descriptive Outcome Report for the last 12 months.
2. Note the differences in the Risk-Adjusted outcomes as compared to the Descriptive outcomes.
3. Highlight those outcomes that have marks (* or **) or (+ or ++) in the significance column.
4. Place a checkmark beside your agency's outcomes that have (* or **) or (+ or ++) as the significance level and at least 30 eligible patient cases.

*Guiding Questions*

- For your agency's outcomes with significance levels at .10 or less and at least 30 Eligible Cases, how does each outcome percentage compare to its corresponding national reference percentage?
- How great is the difference in these percentages?

## CONCEPT APPLICATION:

### Using the Case Mix Profile Report to Give Perspective to the Descriptive Outcome Report

An agency notices that its end result outcome on the Descriptive Outcome Report, *Improvement in Pain Interfering with Activity*, reveals an agency percentage very low in comparison to the national reference average. Asterisks appear in the significance column and have a level of significance at .10. It keeps in mind that while Descriptive Outcomes are worthy of consideration; they have not been risk-adjusted. There are 48 reported cases. The agency reviews its Case Mix Profile Report for the same time period.

In evaluating this outcome, the Case Mix Profile shows that *Terminal Condition* accounted for the highest percentage of *Acute Conditions* and that *Neoplasm* accounted for the highest percentage of home care diagnoses in this same period. This finding from the Case Mix Profile Report gives perspective to the overall evaluation of this outcome. It also gives the agency a more detailed target area. Based on this finding, the agency decides to review a sample of charts of terminal patients with primary diagnosis of Neoplasm to determine the type and quality of care being provided to address patients' pain.

A chart audit tool is developed using recommended interventions from a clinical practice guideline for pain management. The guideline is used as a yardstick to determine the degree to which recommended pain management interventions are ordered by physicians and provided by staff.

**2**B

## AGENCY APPLICATION:

### Using the Case Mix Profile Report to Give Perspective to Outcomes Data

1. Review your agency's Risk Adjusted Outcomes and Descriptive Outcomes Report considering the Case Mix Profile Report for the same time period.
2. Specify any Case Mix Profile descriptors or characteristics that could shed light upon the outcomes that you have checked in the agency application immediately above.

_____

_____

_____

_____

## Patient Tally Reports

There are two OBQI Patient Tally Reports:
1. The Case Mix Tally Report
2. The Outcome Tally Report

The primary use of both reports is to select patients for your outcomes (process of care) investigation. These reports are not typically downloaded until you have targeted an outcome for investigation. Both tally reports list individual patients by name and SOC /ROC date. Patients with multiple SOC/ROC and discharge or transfer assessments will be listed for each episode having occurred during the report period selected for review.

### Case Mix Tally Report

See Figure 2.3 for format of Case Mix Tally Report. For this discussion, also refer to *your agency's* Case Mix Tally Report for the past 12 months. The item numbers used below correspond to the circled numbers in Figure 2.3.

1. **Patient Name** identifies every patient by name included in the report period selected for review.
2. **SOC/ROC Date**—Start of care/Resumption of care date.
3. **Headings** of patient characteristics, such as Demographics, Payment source, and Residence, appearing in the Case Mix Profile Report are also listed in the Case Mix Tally Report.
4. **Patient characteristics** are denoted for each patient as "y" (yes), "n" (no), or "-" (data not available) as entries.
5. A scale **"number"** indicating the patient's OASIS item response, or "–" when no data are available.

**Figure 2.3  Example of Case Mix Tally Report**

| Agency Name: | FAIRCARE HOME HEALTH SERVICES | Medicare Number: | 007001 |
| Agency ID: | HHA01 | Medicaid Number: | 999888001 |
| Location: | ANYTOWN, USA | Date Reported: | 03/21/2003 |

**Case Mix Tally Report**

Report Period: 01/01/2001 12/01/2001

Legend:
y = Attribute present
n = Attribute not present
number = Patient's actual score on item with scale
– = No data collected for this item

| Patient Name | SOC/ROC Date | Age | Gender: Female | Race: Black | Race: White | Race: Other | Any Medicare | Any Medicaid | Any HMO | Medicare HMO | Private Third Party | Own Home | Family member home | Lives alone | With other family member | With friend | With paid help | Spouse/significant other | Daughter/son | Other paid help | No one person | Freq. of assistance (0-6) | From hospital | From rehab facility | From nursing home | Medical regimen change | Moderate recovery prognosis | Good rehab prognosis |
|---|---|---|---|---|---|---|---|---|---|---|---|---|---|---|---|---|---|---|---|---|---|---|---|---|---|---|---|---|
| | | | | | | | Payment Source | | | | | Residence | | Current Living Situation | | | | Primary Caretaker | | | | | Inpt DC | | | Med Heg | Prognoses | |
| ANDERSON, -------- | 06/12/01 | 74 | y | n | y | n | y | n | n | n | n | y | n | y | n | n | n | n | n | n | n | y | 0 | y | n | n | n | y | y |
| BROWN, ----------- | 11/24/00 | 66 | y | n | y | n | y | y | n | n | n | y | n | y | n | n | n | n | n | n | y | 0 | n | n | n | n | y | y | y |
| BYRNNE, ----------- | 08/24/01 | 81 | y | n | y | n | y | n | n | n | n | n | n | n | n | n | y | n | n | y | n | y | n | 5 | n | n | n | n | y | y |

## AGENCY APPLICATION:
### Reading the Case Mix Tally Report

1. Review your agency's Case Mix Tally Report for the last 12 months.
2. Note number of patient cases generated.
3. Familiarize yourself with each component of the report.
4. Place your Case Mix Tally Report alongside the Case Mix Profile Report for the same report period. Note similarities and differences of both reports.
5. From your agency's Case Mix Profile Report, select one category that you previously highlighted that displays (* or **) or (+ or ++) of significance. There may be more than one characteristic in the category with asterisks. Select one characteristic.
6. Locate this category and the characteristic on your agency's Case Mix Tally Report. Note the patients who have or who do not have the characteristic.

### Guiding Questions

- Do I understand the significance of the Case Mix Tally Report?
- Do I know when to generate a Case Mix Tally Report?

**2**B

## Outcome Tally Report

See Figure 2.4 for format of Outcome Tally Report. The item numbers used below correspond to the circled numbers in Figure 2.4.

For this discussion, refer to *your agency's* Outcome Tally Report for the past 12 months. (This 12-month report will be lengthy because all patients' outcomes are included.)

1. **Patient Name** identifies every patient by name that is included in the report period selected for review.
2. **SOC/ROC Date**.
3. **Headings** of Health Status Outcomes and Utilization Outcomes.
4. **Health Status** or **End Result Outcomes** are noted for each patient as:

   - "x" – the patient achieved the outcome
   - "o" – the patient did not achieve the outcome
   - "-" – the outcome could not be calculated

5. **Utilization outcomes** are denoted as:

   - "y" – yes, the service was utilized
   - "n" – no, the service was not utilized

## Figure 2.4 Example of Outcome Tally Report

| | |
|---|---|
| Agency Name: FAIRCARE HOME HEALTH SERVICES | Medicare Number: 007001 |
| Agency ID: HHA01 | Medicaid Number: 999888001 |
| Location: ANYTOWN, USA | Date Reported: 02/28/2002 |

### Outcome Tally Report

Report Period: 01/01/2001-12/01/2001 — Health Status Outcomes / Utilization Outcomes

Legend:
x = Patient achieved outcome
o = Patient did not achieve outcome
– = Outcome not computed for patient
y = Yes
n = No

| Patient Name | SOC/ROC Date | Improv in speech or language | Stabil in speech or language | Improv in pain interfering with activity | Improv in number of surgical wounds | Improv in status surgical wounds | Improv in dyspnea | Improv in urinary tract infection | Improv in urinary incontinence | Improv in behavioral problem frequency | Improv in bowel incontinence | Improv in cognitive functioning | Improv in confusion frequency | Improv in anxiety level | Stabil in anxiety level | Improv in behavioral problem frequency | Discharged to the community | Acute care hospitalization | Improv in behavioral problem frequency |
|---|---|---|---|---|---|---|---|---|---|---|---|---|---|---|---|---|---|---|---|
| ANDERSON, -------- | 06/12/01 | – | x | o | x | o | o | – | o | – | – | x | – | – | o | – | n | y | n |
| BROWN, ------------ | 11/24/00 | – | x | – | – | – | x | – | – | – | – | x | – | – | x | – | n | y | n |
| BYRNNE, ----------- | 08/24/01 | o | o | x | – | – | x | – | – | – | o | x | o | – | x | – | n | y | n |

This report contains confidential information to be used only by the Home Health Agency and State Agency and is not to be shared with any other individuals, in accordance with 42 CFR 484.11 Condition of Participation: Release of patient identifiable info.

OBQI Implementation Manual 02/2002 A.13

---

## AGENCY APPLICATION:
## Reading the Outcome Tally Report

1. Review your agency's Outcome Tally Report for the last 12 months.
2. Note number of patients generated.
3. Familiarize yourself with each component of the report.
4. Place your Outcome Tally Report alongside your Risk-Adjusted and Descriptive Outcomes Report for the same time period. Note the similarities and differences.
5. From your agency's Risk-Adjusted and Descriptive Outcomes Report, select one outcome that you previously highlighted that displays (* or **) or (+ or ++) of significance.
6. Locate this outcome on your agency's Outcome Tally Report. Note the patients who achieved and did not achieve the outcome.

### Guiding Questions

- Do I understand the purpose of the Outcome Tally Report?
- Do I know when to generate an Outcome Tally Report?

## A Workbook Tool to Facilitate the Use of Tally Reports

Agencies can use a Microsoft Excel workbook, a software tool that enhances data import from the Case Mix and Outcome Tally Reports and is downloaded from CASPER (the same software used to send OASIS data to the state) in a spreadsheet format (Crisler and Richard, 2003). The spreadsheet produced by the workbook tool is in the **same format** as that of the Patient Tally Reports.

The tool automates the process of selecting specific patient cases and episodes to review based on patient outcome and/or case mix characteristics (Crisler and Richard, 2003). This workbook tool helps the agency refine patient episodes and cases to a manageable number. The tool enables the agency to:

1. run a query according to the outcome name and whether or not the outcome was achieved for selected episodes, and to
2. run additional queries of case mix characteristics that can be applied to outcome findings for selected episodes (Crisler and Richard, 2003).

*When running a query according to the outcome and whether or not the outcome was achieved*, you select one or more outcomes. However, to be included in your query results, the patient must meet all of your selection criteria. For example, if you want to know which patients did not achieve the outcomes of *Improvement in bathing* and *Improvement in dressing upper body*, your query results will yield only those episodes for patients meeting both criteria of:

- not achieving the outcome of *Improvement in bathing,* **and**
- not achieving the outcome of I*mprovement in upper body dressing.*

Note that the fewer queries you run, the greater the number of episodes and cases the tool will produce. For example, if you run a query only of those not showing an *Improvement in bathing,* the potential result of this query alone is hundreds of episodes and cases.

Running additional queries of outcomes and/or case mix characteristics can narrow this number. When running additional queries for case mix characteristics, refer to the outcome(s) in question. For instance, in the previous example we queried patients **not** having *Improvement in bathing,* **and not** having *Improvement in upper body dressing.*

For example, your initial query of patients who did not improve in bathing and dressing upper body yields multiple episodes. Subsequent to this, you run additional queries of race, gender, financial factors, limited or no assistance, and those living alone, for these same episodes. Running these additional queries helps you to narrow the number of patients who are included in your outcomes investigation. Of course, clinical judgment is needed to select queries that are appropriate to the patient outcomes in question.

---

### AGENCY APPLICATION:

### Using the Workbook Tool to Select Outcome and Case Mix Queries

*Note: It is recommended that you refer to the CMS OASIS website at http://www.cms.hhs.gov/oasis/obqi.asp for current software and system requirements, the latest revision of the workbook tool, and its current instructions for use.*

Before you can use the workbook tool, you must:

1. Save both your Case Mix Tally Report and your Outcomes Tally Report in spreadsheet format to a folder on your hard drive. (Date range for both reports MUST be the same.)
2. Download the CMSTallyTemplate.xls and instructions for use (from the CMS website address) to your hard drive.
3. Print the accompanying instructions entitled: *Instructions for Working with the Patient Tally Report Workbook Template.*

## AGENCY APPLICATION:
### Using the Workbook Tool to Select Outcome and Case Mix Queries *(continued)*

4. Follow the Workbook Tool instructions to select the following OASIS outcome criteria by name for patients who *did not meet the outcomes* of:
   * Improvement in pain interfering with activity
   * Improvement in bathing
   * Improvement in dressing upper body
   * Improvement in dressing lower body
5. Note the number of cases this query produced.
6. Select the following Case Mix Criteria and apply them to the patient cases above, to obtain a single patient group.
   *14. Dyspnea*
   *23. Diagnosis for Home Care: Respiratory*
7. Note the number of patient episodes and cases that the Case Mix query yielded.

These queries generated a patient group that has dyspnea and a respiratory diagnosis who *did not improve* in the outcomes of bathing, dressing upper and lower body, or pain interfering with activity. Using these patient characteristics, you can now conduct a focused chart review for your outcomes (process of care) investigation.

### Guiding Questions

* Has your query yielded a manageable size of patient cases for review and investigation?
* What does your chart review reveal about the care provided to this patient group?
* Are usual interventions provided? What are the similarities and differences in this patient group that could account for less than desired outcomes?
* Do best practice interventions exist for pain management and/or respiratory care? If so, are these interventions appropriate and reasonable for your patient population? Do the interventions address the outcomes you desire?
* Are there additional queries that would make this investigation more meaningful for this patient group?

# Adverse Event Outcome Report for OBQM

This report reflects potential problems in care because of their negative nature. Whether or not an individual patient outcome is a consequence of inadequate care can be determined only through an investigation of the care actually provided to the patient (HCFA, 2001).

As of this writing, the Adverse Event Outcomes are:

- Emergent care for injury caused by fall or accident at home
- Emergent care for wound infections, deteriorating wound status
- Emergent care for improper medication administration, medication side effects
- Emergent care for hypo/hyperglycemia
- Development of urinary tract infection
- Increase in number of pressure ulcers
- Substantial decline in three or more ADLs
- Substantial decline in management of oral medications
- Unexpected nursing home admission
- Discharged to the community needing wound care or medication assistance
- Discharged to the community needing toileting assistance
- Discharged to the community with behavioral problems
- Unexpected death

Consider OASIS data set items:
MO450:          Current number of pressure ulcers at each stage
MO830/MO840:  Emergent care; Emergent care reason #5: wound infection, deteriorating wound status, new lesion/ulcer

Answers to *MO450* & *MO830/MO840*, over OASIS assessment *time points* during the length of service, generate outcomes for patients who have had a pressure ulcer or who have required emergent care for a wound. These outcomes are aggregated into a percentage on the OBQM Adverse Event Outcome Report as:

*Emergent care for wound infections, deteriorating wound status %.*
*Increase in number of Pressure Ulcers %.*

## Report Format and Description

See Figure 2.5 for format of Adverse Event Outcome Report. The following item numbers correspond to the circled numbers in Figure 2.5. For this discussion, also refer to your agency's Adverse Event Outcome Report for the past 12 months.

1. The **first column** to the left of the page lists the adverse event **outcomes by name**.
2. The **second column** gives the number of **patient cases** in the report period. There are two numbers in this column. The top number reflects the agency's number of patient cases, and the bottom number represents the national reference number of cases.
3. The **third column** is **Signif. (significance)**. Asterisks that appear in the significance column on this report indicate that the difference between the agency's outcome and the national reference has a 90–95% probability of being real, not due to chance.
4. The **fourth column** has **Bar Graphs** that indicate the percentage of patients who experienced the adverse event. The white bar represents the agency's current percentage of patients. The dark shaded bar represents the national reference percentage.

## Figure 2.5  Example of Adverse Event Outcome Report

**Agency Name: FAIRCARE HOME HEALTH SERVICES**
**Agency ID: HHA01**
**Location: ANYTOWN, USA**
**Medicare Number: 007001**
**Medicare Number: 999888001**

**Requested Current Period: 09/1999 - 08/2000**
**Actual Current Period: 09/1999 - 08/2000**
**Number of Cases in Current Period: 601**
**Number of Cases in Reference Sample: 29983**
**Date Report Printed: 11/30/2000**

### Adverse Event Outcome Report

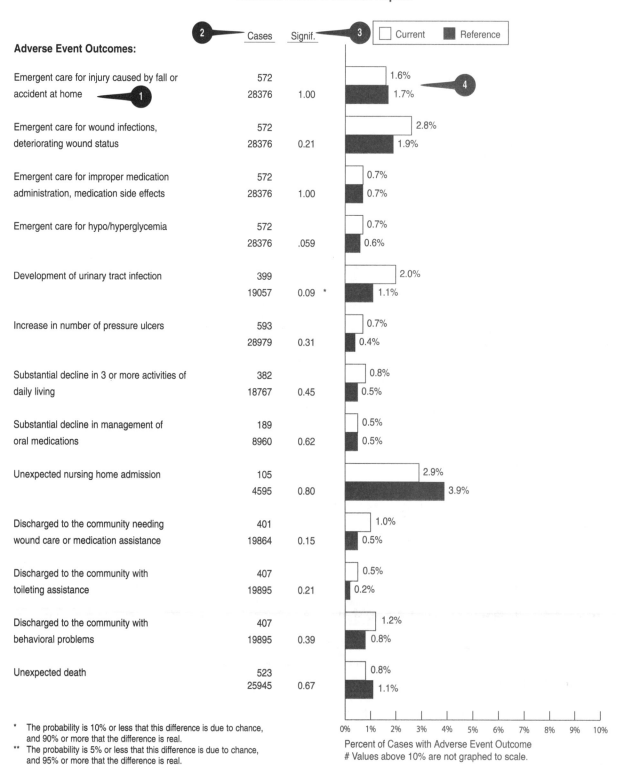

| Adverse Event Outcomes: | Cases | Signif. | | |
|---|---|---|---|---|
| | | | □ Current | ■ Reference |
| Emergent care for injury caused by fall or accident at home | 572 28376 | 1.00 | 1.6% | 1.7% |
| Emergent care for wound infections, deteriorating wound status | 572 28376 | 0.21 | 2.8% | 1.9% |
| Emergent care for improper medication administration, medication side effects | 572 28376 | 1.00 | 0.7% | 0.7% |
| Emergent care for hypo/hyperglycemia | 572 28376 | .059 | 0.7% | 0.6% |
| Development of urinary tract infection | 399 19057 | 0.09 * | 2.0% | 1.1% |
| Increase in number of pressure ulcers | 593 28979 | 0.31 | 0.7% | 0.4% |
| Substantial decline in 3 or more activities of daily living | 382 18767 | 0.45 | 0.8% | 0.5% |
| Substantial decline in management of oral medications | 189 8960 | 0.62 | 0.5% | 0.5% |
| Unexpected nursing home admission | 105 4595 | 0.80 | 2.9% | 3.9% |
| Discharged to the community needing wound care or medication assistance | 401 19864 | 0.15 | 1.0% | 0.5% |
| Discharged to the community with toileting assistance | 407 19895 | 0.21 | 0.5% | 0.2% |
| Discharged to the community with behavioral problems | 407 19895 | 0.39 | 1.2% | 0.8% |
| Unexpected death | 523 25945 | 0.67 | 0.8% | 1.1% |

\*   The probability is 10% or less that this difference is due to chance, and 90% or more that the difference is real.
\*\* The probability is 5% or less that this difference is due to chance, and 95% or more that the difference is real.

0%   1%   2%   3%   4%   5%   6%   7%   8%   9%   10%
Percent of Cases with Adverse Event Outcome
# Values above 10% are not graphed to scale.

## AGENCY APPLICATION:
## Reading the Adverse Event Outcome Report

1. Using your agency's Adverse Event Outcome Report for the last 12 months, locate the following outcomes:
   - *Emergent care for wound infection, deteriorating wound status,* and
   - *Increase in number of pressure ulcers.*

   Do you see asterisks of significance for either outcome? _____

2. If so, highlight these. What is the relevance that this outcome has to your agency's patient population?

   _____

   _____

   _____

3. Using this same OASIS Adverse Event Outcome Report, highlight *all* of your agency's outcomes that have asterisks in the significance column. Of these, which outcomes have the greatest clinical relevance to the patients you serve?

   _____

   _____

**2**B

## Figure 2.6  Example of Adverse Event Outcome Report—Patient Listing

Agency Name: FAIRCARE HOME HEALTH SERVICES
Agency ID: HHA01
Location: ANYTOWN, USA
Medicare Number: 007001
Medicare Number: 999888001

Requested Current Period: 09/1999 - 08/2000
Actual Current Period: 09/1999 - 08/2000
Number of Cases in Current Period: 601
Number of Cases in Reference Sample: 29983
Date Report Printed: 11/30/2000

### Adverse Event Outcome Report
#### Patient Listing

### Development of Urinary Tract Infection

Complete Data Cases:  399         Number of Events:  8         Agency Incidence:  2.0%         Reference Incidence:  1.1%

| Patient ID | Last Name | First Name | Gender | Birth Date | SOC/ROC | DC/Transfer |
|---|---|---|---|---|---|---|
| 859294045 | Dunn | Jim | M | 10/17/1920 | 11/20/99 | 12/19/99 |
| 565570409 | Rosling | Walter | M | 10/21/1938 | 05/26/00 | 08/13/00 |
| 014760252 | Connelly | Sherwood | M | 11/14/1940 | 07/29/00 | 08/30/00 |
| 472551333 | Guinn | Rosemary | F | 08/18/1915 | 03/17/00 | 03/26/00 |
| 773642368 | Mullins | Caleb | M | 01/23/1938 | 10/19/99 | 01/20/00 |
| 759333066 | Beck | Jan | F | 07/04/1929 | 07/25/00 | 07/30/00 |
| 136056137 | Hayes | Edd | M | 10/05/1929 | 05/07/00 | 05/07/00 |
| 947917397 | St. Germain | Teri | F | 11/29/1940 | 06/17/00 | 07/18/00 |

### Increase in Number of Pressure Ulcers

Complete Data Cases:  593         Number of Events:  4         Agency Incidence:  0.7%         Reference Incidence:  0.4%

| Patient ID | Last Name | First Name | Gender | Birth Date | SOC/ROC | DC/Transfer |
|---|---|---|---|---|---|---|
| 315867385 | Dodge | Robert | M | 12/06/1937 | 10/29/99 | 11/09/99 |
| 133711082 | Koch | Jane | F | 11/11/1915 | 10/20/99 | 02/14/00 |
| 417495912 | Beal | Tracy | F | 04/07/1914 | 04/05/00 | 07/06/00 |
| 870032669 | Martineau | Lyn | M | 12/19/1930 | 07/24/00 | 08/03/00 |

### Substantial Decline in 3 or More Activities of Daily Living

Complete Data Cases:  382         Number of Events:  3         Agency Incidence:  0.8%         Reference Incidence:  0.5%

| Patient ID | Last Name | First Name | Gender | Birth Date | SOC/ROC | DC/Transfer |
|---|---|---|---|---|---|---|
| 854314071 | Henrich | Byron | M | 06/29/1940 | 04/06/00 | 08/02/00 |
| 424787337 | Seals | Flo | F | 11/20/1927 | 02/01/00 | 02/21/00 |
| 500582191 | Klebe | Kathleen | F | 08/26/1916 | 01/27/00 | 04/03/00 |

### Substantial Decline in Management of Oral Medications

Complete Data Cases:  189         Number of Events:  1         Agency Incidence:  0.5%         Reference Incidence:  0.5%

| Patient ID | Last Name | First Name | Gender | Birth Date | SOC/ROC | DC/Transfer |
|---|---|---|---|---|---|---|
| 502513146 | Botello | Brenda | F | 06/03/1924 | 05/01/00 | 08/20/00 |

### Unexpected Nursing Home Admission

Complete Data Cases:  105         Number of Events:  3         Agency Incidence:  2.9%         Reference Incidence:  3.9%

| Patient ID | Last Name | First Name | Gender | Birth Date | SOC/ROC | DC/Transfer |
|---|---|---|---|---|---|---|
| 952821056 | Burcham | Nancy | F | 09/17/1936 | 05/30/00 | 07/08/00 |
| 118840231 | Elder | Jean | F | 01/20/1923 | 09/06/99 | 10/15/99 |
| 645083076 | Condon | Jack | M | 04/29/1929 | 07/20/00 | 08/05/00 |

## Adverse Event Outcome Report—Patient Listing

Patients' individual identifying information appears on the report titled: Adverse Event Outcome Report—Patient Listing. This is available for further investigation of each patient's case as needed, and for chart review. The report lists each Adverse Event Outcome with the names of all patients having experienced each outcome in the report period.

See Figure 2.6 for format of Adverse Event Outcome Report—Patient Listing. The item numbers used below correspond to the circled numbers in Figure 2.6. For this discussion, refer to your agency's Adverse Event Outcome Report—Patient Listing for the past 12 months.

1. **Complete Data Cases** (patient cases).
2. **Number of events** that occurred in the time period.
3. **Agency incidence** (agency percentage having occurred in the time period).
4. **Reference incidence** (national percentage having occurred in the time period).
5. **Patient ID**.
6. **Patient's last name**.
7. **Patient's first name**.
8. **Patient's gender**.
9. **Patient's birth date**.
10. **SOC/ROC date**.
11. **Patient D/C/Transfer date**.

2B

---

### AGENCY APPLICATION:

### Reading the Adverse Event Report: Patient Listing

1. Place your agency's Adverse Event Outcome Report alongside your Adverse Event Outcome—Patient Listing for the same time period.

2. Note the highlighted outcomes that you checked on the Adverse Event Outcome Report in the previous application.

3. Locate these outcomes in the Adverse Event Outcome Report—Patient Listing.

4. Note the number of events (patient cases) for each.

*Note: OBQM suggests that if 30 cases are listed for the Adverse Event, at least 20 cases be reviewed. If less than 20 cases are listed, all cases should be reviewed.

---

## AGENCY APPLICATION:

### Using the Case Mix Profile Report to Give Perspective to the Adverse Event Outcome Report

An agency's Adverse Event Outcome Report reveals percentages that are well above the national reference for the following outcomes, and have asterisks indicating the probability that the difference in the outcomes is not due to chance:

- *Increase in number of pressure ulcers*
- *Emergent care for wound infections, deteriorating wound status*

The Case Mix Report, which is inclusive of the dates of the Adverse Event Report, has been run. The following characteristics were taken from the agency's Case Mix Profile Report and summarized here. The summary reveals the following percentages in relation to the national reference average that have asterisks of significance on the report:

| *Characteristics* | *Agency Case Mix* | *National Reference* |
|---|---|---|
| Average age (in years): | 79 yrs | 73 yrs |
| Integumentary Status: Pressure ulcer(s) | 14% | 9% |
| Elimination Status: Urinary Incontinence | 12% | 8% |
| Chronic conditions: Chronic patient with caretaker | 41% | 33% |
| Current Living Situation: Lives Alone | 20% | 14% |
| Primary Caretaker: No one person | 33% | 26% |
| Home Care Diagnoses: Skin/Subcutaneous diseases | 10.8% | 6.7% |

When clinical judgment is used to review these factors collectively, perspective is gained into possible causes. As the agency prepares for a thorough investigation that includes chart review and employee interview, what are some of the possible causes they should keep in mind?

_____

_____

_____

_____

*Answer: Possible causes include the higher-than-average pressure ulcer population that is close to 80 years of age with a predisposing skin condition. The increase in urinary incontinence can easily be a contributing factor to pressure ulcer development and wound deterioration. A large percentage of this patient group lives alone, with no one primary caretaker; this setting makes an aggressive and focused daily treatment plan difficult to carry out.*

# SELECTING OASIS OUTCOMES FOR REVIEW & PI

Because an outcome-based approach to care will likely impact agency work processes, staff development, and resource utilization, agency leadership must be involved in reviewing outcome reports, and in selecting or approving outcomes that the agency will *target* for investigation. OBQI allows each agency to determine which outcomes are investigated and how to address outcomes significantly below national benchmarks. The agency also determines the appropriate best practices to implement based on the OASIS outcomes achieved. Performance improvement methods and tools are used to positively impact end-result outcomes.

You must keep certain criteria in mind as you evaluate your OASIS outcome reports to determine outcomes that need to be addressed to enhance quality of care or to reinforce care being given (CMS, 2002). The method used to select outcomes for investigation in OBQI is somewhat different than that for OBQM. The criteria for each are listed below.

*Note: Some material already mentioned will be briefly reiterated here, as its importance bears repeating.*

2B

## Selecting Target Outcomes in OBQI

Select and prioritize your OASIS *target* outcomes from the OBQI Risk-Adjusted and Descriptive Outcome Report by evaluating them in this order:

1. Highlight those having asterisks in the **significance** column.
2. Consider the **magnitude of the difference** in the agency and the reference outcome percentages. For example, a difference of five percentage points is less important than a difference of sixteen.
3. Note the **number of cases** reported for each outcome. The outcome should have at least 30 cases reported in order for it to be considered a target outcome for investigation, regardless of its significance. A small number of cases can result in a large percentage change in the outcome. A larger sample size minimizes this.
4. Note the difference in the **levels of significance** reported. *Select those outcomes with significance less than or equal to .10.* If no outcomes meet the criteria, note those that are closest to .10 and no greater than .25. Disregard outcomes with levels of significance greater than .25.
5. After completing steps 1–4, highlight those outcomes that have particular relevance to your agency's overall goals. Consider these in light of your agency case mix, payer mix, agency goals, and strategic plan. Also consider outcomes that have clinical significance in the provision of care. These may be diagnoses, conditions, or interventions:

   - of high volume
   - that tend to be problematic
   - of high cost and increased resource utilization
   - where clinical quality is an issue

## Monitoring Outcomes in OBQM

1. Review the overall content of your agency's Adverse Event Outcomes Report.
2. Note those outcomes having asterisks in the significance column and at least those with a higher incidence than the national reference.
3. Review the agency's Case Mix Profile Report in depth.
4. Note those areas that have asterisks of significance, but do not limit your review and evaluation of the report based on these alone. Ascertain the overall picture of your patient population, relative to the Adverse Event Outcomes.
5. Of these outcomes, prioritize and select those for investigation first that have the

greatest clinical relevance to the care provided, and those with the highest incidence as compared to the reference group. Ideally, the Adverse Event Outcome(s)
you select first for investigation will meet both criteria (HCFA, 2001).

6. Review all patient cases for the outcome(s) in question.

---

### AGENCY APPLICATION:
### Selecting Outcomes for Investigation

1. From the previous review and highlighting of your agency's outcome reports, use the criteria above to select one or two OBQI target outcomes for actual investigation. List these from your Risk-Adjusted and Descriptive Outcome Report:

_____

_____

_____

_____

_____

2. From criteria given for prioritizing outcomes in OBQM, select outcomes you will investigate first from your Adverse Event Outcome Report:

_____

_____

_____

_____

_____

---

## ANALYSIS AND INVESTIGATION OF OASIS OUTCOMES DATA

Even though outcomes can be measured, aggregated, analyzed, and interpreted in a variety of ways, the subsequent investigation of outcomes data is basically conducted through the framework of performance improvement. OBQI recommends outcomes analysis and investigation be conducted at least quarterly. While the following steps are outlined sequentially, they can be undertaken simultaneously.

*Step 1—Designate a member of leadership to facilitate outcomes evaluation, interpretation, and analysis.*

- Involve the agency's leadership team throughout the process.
- Involve clinical staff in the process through a focus group, PI team, chart review, feedback, and/or brainstorming.

*Step 2—Verify the accuracy of your outcomes data.*

- Are staff using correct OASIS response instructions when assessing patients? (Conduct clinical data audits, written or oral competencies, or make *side-by-side* home visits with clinicians.)
- Is Data Entry correctly keying in OASIS documentation provided by clinicians? (Conduct periodic Data Entry Audits to determine the percentage of keying error.)

*Step 3—Review outcome reports to get an overall sense of the content.*

*Step 4—Review demographics specifically for your patient population during the same time period that care is provided.*

- Give perspective to these outcome percentages.
- Review the Case Mix Profile Report in light of outcomes you have highlighted on the Risk-Adjusted and Descriptive Outcome Report and the Adverse Event Outcome Report.

*Step 5—Choose one or two OBQI target outcomes that appear to need remediation or reinforcement, and prioritize the Adverse Event outcomes that will be investigated first.*

*Step 6—Evaluate existing care by establishing best practice standards of care that should be provided to patients related to the OBQI target outcome(s) (Crisler and Richard, 2002c).*

These can be ascertained through professional expertise, a review of published literature or other health-related research, and policy and procedure. For example, let's say that the agency has an Adverse Event priority outcome of an *Increase in the number of pressure ulcers*. How does the agency's level of care for a patient with a pressure ulcer compare to best practices that are recommended for improvement of outcomes? The agency may also have a policy and procedure that outlines other aspects of pressure ulcer care.

In another example, an agency has a standard of care for fall prevention. If the Adverse Event outcome being addressed is *Emergent care for injury caused by fall or accident at home,* the agency will use its best practice standard of care for fall prevention as the yardstick by which this aspect of care will be investigated.

By contrast, an agency may not have a standard of care and chooses to develop one based on unacceptable outcomes. For example, an agency has a higher percentage of patients with falls and injury requiring emergent care. It decides to develop a best practice standard for fall and injury prevention designed to improve this outcome.

*Step 7—Determine the likely cause of the outcome(s) needing remediation or reinforcement.*

Specify the approach(es) that will be used to investigate the clinical aspects of care that are provided to patients. Staff interviews? Meeting discussions? Questionnaire? Reviews of staff competency? Home Visit Observation? Medical record review?

## Guiding Questions

- Does the agency provide care according to the standard, best practices, or policy and procedure?
- If so, are staff running into obstacles as they implement care according to established standards?
- Do the staff know the standard?

- Do one or more elements of the standard need revision?
- Does a tool need to be developed to conduct a questionnaire or guide interviews.
- Does a special chart review tool need to be designed to review care? To tally results? Who will devise these tools?

### Selecting Medical Records for Review

Use the Case Mix Profile Report and the Patient Outcome Tally Report or the Adverse Event Outcome—Patient Listing to select individual patient medical records for review. Use the workbook tool in OBQI as necessary to derive a manageable number of cases. *OBQI suggests that 30 records be reviewed* for targeted outcome investigation (CMS, 2002).

In the investigation of an adverse event outcome, DHHS (2001) suggests the review of at least 20 cases if more than 30 are in the total listing. If fewer than 30 cases are listed for each adverse event, every case should be investigated.

- Develop a chart review tool as needed that includes the best practices you have outlined in *Step 6*.
- Determine the portion of the episode necessary for review.
- Conduct the review by comparing care rendered to best practice recommendations.
- Aggregate results.

### Step 8—Summarize findings.

- Review aggregated findings from all sources.
- List all aspects of care discovered from staff interviews, chart reviews, home visit observation, financial reviews, and other agency documentation that seemed to be problematic and that have the greatest potential for improving the OASIS selected outcomes.
- Now state these in specific detail. For example:
  - Only 30% of all staff can verbalize the elements of the agency's fall prevention guideline.
  - The agency's fall prevention guideline is distributed to only 50% of all patients 70 years of age and older on admission. Policy states that all patients 70 and older will receive fall prevention guideline.
  - The agency does not use a specific risk assessment tool for pressure ulcer prevention.
  - Agency costs exceed reimbursement for treatment of pressure ulcers 72% of the time.
- Apply graphs, charts, and/or PI methods and tools (Joint Commission, 1994) to help prioritize findings.
- Select aspects of care delivery that need to be changed to improve outcomes or those that need to be reinforced to maintain desired outcomes.

### Step 9—Develop a plan of action.

- Appoint an individual to facilitate writing the plan. Keep it simple.
- Identify the problem(s) in statement form.
- Appoint clinically qualified individuals to review best practice recommendations, and to revise, or write new standards or processes.
- Write these in the form of statements.
- Determine what resources, if any, are needed to implement best practices.
- Determine what must occur to procure these resources.
- Outline components of staff education required to implement new or revised care processes. Will staff need new or additional skills and competencies? When will this training take place? Who will provide training? Where will training take place? On-site, off-site?

- Include new processes and competencies in new employee orientation.
- Determine how and when all remaining staff will be informed of these findings and of the implementation date of the new or revised standards, guidelines and policy, and procedure.

### Step 10—Implement best practice recommendations or standards of care.

As appropriate, discuss a best practice recommendation of care with the agency Medical Director or Advisor.

*Note: When an agency adopts a particular standard of care for a patient diagnosis, condition, or situation, the patient's physician must approve the intervention for it to become a part of the POC.*

*Note: Until changes are made in care delivery, undesired outcomes are likely to remain unchanged. Crisler and Richard (2002a) recommend that a plan of action begin within one month of obtaining the outcomes report.*

### Step 11—Perform implementation follow-up.

- Perform follow-up as early as two weeks of implementation to determine if directives are being implemented.
- Get feedback from management and clinical staff through interviews, staff meeting discussions, home visit follow-up, and case conferences.
- Conduct follow-up medical record review as necessary, and at least quarterly.
- Review OBQI/OBQM Outcome reports on at least a quarterly basis to determine the trend of target outcome percentages.
- Provide detailed follow-up feedback to all management and clinical staff on a regular basis.
- Reinforce acceptable outcomes achieved and continue to investigate and improve those that are unacceptable. *This is the cycle that forms the basis of performance improvement.*
- Celebrate successes with staff!

---

### CONCEPT APPLICATION:

### Developing Best Practices in Response to an OASIS Adverse Event Outcome(s) Investigation

An agency has recurring problems with the following OASIS outcomes:

- *Increase in number of pressure ulcers*
- *Emergent care for wound infections, deteriorating wound status*

The agency has completed a full investigation of what is potentially contributing to these less than desired outcomes. The agency reviewed the OASIS Case Mix Profile Report based on these outcomes, as well as its own financial reports regarding cost, reimbursement, visits, and supplies.

The agency completed other activities related to this investigation—a medical record review of a large sample of patients (taken from the Adverse Event—Patient Listing), staff interviews, and home visit observations with both skilled staff and home health aides.

## CONCEPT APPLICATION:

### Developing Best Practices in Response to an OASIS Adverse Event Outcome(s) Investigation *(continued)*

An excerpt from the summary of the investigation revealed the following problem statements:

- A majority of patients appearing on the OASIS Adverse Event Patient Listing had a primary diagnosis of pressure ulcer.
- The OASIS Case Mix Profile indicated a high percentage of Stage 3–4 pressure ulcers.
- One third of these patients had no one caretaker or lived alone.
- The supply room had many different varieties of wound products on the shelves.
- Nurses were unsure when to recommend a change in treatment to the physician.
- Some nurses were unsure of how to properly stage an ulcer.
- Nutrition for promotion of healing was not consistently addressed in majority of cases.
- Home health aides provided usual care specific to skin inspection and skin care needs of this patient population.
- Therapists were involved only 25% of the time for patients who had problems with transferring.
- The agency had no wound specialty nurse accessible to staff for consultation.
- The risk assessment tool in place was completed 98% of the time on admission. However, 60% of these assessments had no evidence of continued follow-up.

Because of the multiplicity of findings in the agency's investigation, leadership decides that implementing best practice recommendations is best to improve these outcomes. The agency first researches a clinical practice guideline for the patient with pressure ulcer. It also reviews its cost including supply utilization versus reimbursement. It determines that additional agency supplemental outcomes need to be developed and measured.

The following is an *excerpt* of the standards of care designed by the agency to address problems that could be adversely affecting the outcomes of its patients with a primary diagnosis of pressure ulcer:

Primary Diagnosis:
Pressure Ulcer

### Agency Best Practice Statements (Standards of Care) (excerpt):

- All adult patients will have the XYZ pressure ulcer risk assessment completed on admission visit.
- Patients scoring "X" on risk assessment will be evaluated for a pressure reduction device appropriate to needs.
- If wound is not showing signs of improvement within two weeks of any treatment change, notify physician.
- Agency ABC teaching handout, *Nutrition for Wound Healing*, will be used for patient education and will be taken to the residence on admission or by the second visit.

# CONCEPT APPLICATION:

## Developing Best Practices in Response to an OASIS Adverse Event Outcome(s) Investigation *(continued)*

**Agency Best Practice Statements (Standards of Care) (excerpt continued):**

- Patients with a diagnosis of pressure ulcer and a response of two-to-four for OASIS *MO690: Transferring* and/or response of two-to-three for *MO680: Toileting* will be considered for Physical Therapy evaluation.
- Home Health Aide will massage bony prominences with patient's choice of body cream or lotion. Pressure reduction is applied as appropriate to situation. (Specified in Home Health Aide assignment.)
- Patients over 65 years old with a response of "no one caretaker" or "lives alone" for OASIS *MO360* will be evaluated further for appropriateness of care setting and primary caretaker responsibility.

Other agency interventions:

1. Availability of wound specialty consultation will be researched.
2. Staff education for nursing will include pressure ulcer staging, nutrition to promote healing, use of wound products, and pressure reduction. Home Health Aide education will include types of pressure reduction and how to achieve maximum pressure relief.
3. Staff competency will include staging of pressure ulcers.
4. Product lines will be re-evaluated. Multi-product inventory will be reduced to no more than two complete product lines; miscellaneous items will be ordered if physician feels that current product line will not yield same results.

The following is an excerpt of Agency Selected Outcomes:

OASIS outcomes:

- Increase in the number of pressure ulcers.
- Emergent care for wound infections, deteriorating wound status.

Agency Supplemental Outcomes:

Going forward from this investigation, the agency will measure its own supplemental outcomes relative to pressure ulcer in addition to OASIS outcome measures. These are:

- Patient/caretaker verbalizes signs and symptoms of infection/deterioration by visit six.
- Patient/caretaker demonstrates effective pressure reduction by visit three.
- Patient/caretaker compliant with utilizing effective pressure reduction by visit four.
- Patient/caretaker verbalizes proper food intake to promote wound healing by visit five.

**2**B

■ NOTES ■

## INTEGRATING OASIS OUTCOMES DATA INTO CLINICAL PRACTICE

Some agencies misguidedly think that because they complete and transmit OASIS data set items and review OASIS outcome reports that they are integrating outcomes into clinical practice. While these are important steps, it is only the beginning. While some agencies struggle with staff accuracy of OASIS outcome measurements, others are somewhat unsure of which performance improvement methods to use to improve care provision.

In the Summary Report on OASIS and OBQI in Home Healthcare, Shaugnessy, Crisler, Hittle, and Schlenker (2002) recognized that significant problems had occurred from either 1) inadequate attention to efficiently integrating OASIS into day-to-day assessment and data collection routines of clinical staff or 2) technically flawed or inefficient implementation of systems for computerizing and transmitting OASIS data.

As state surveyors provide feedback on agency progress with the implementation of OBQI, and as agency outcome reports are compared and published, other evaluations of outcomes integration can be anticipated.

To fully integrate OASIS outcomes data into clinical practice, an agency must:

- Accurately document patient responses to OASIS items according to definition.
- Ensure accurate OASIS data entry.
- Transmit OASIS data according to acceptable timeframes.
- Properly review OASIS outcome reports.
- Select target outcomes for investigation.
- Implement clinical processes and strategies with timeliness to improve outcomes.
- Demonstrate improvement in outcomes selected for remediation or demonstrate sustained or enhanced improvement of those outcomes selected for reinforcement.

Successful integration of OASIS outcomes into clinical practice requires the commitment of agency leadership. Setting the stage for change is challenging, but certain key factors have been identified as contributors to success in modifying care delivery (HCFA, 2001). While these things seem obvious, many times they do not receive proper attention.

1. Explain the reason for the transition to outcome based-quality improvement to all staff. Periodic repetition of new and complex information is necessary for forming new habits.
2. Educate staff to new skills and information that will be required of them. All staff are affected by OASIS outcomes information and data in different ways. The skilled disciplines of RN, RPT, OT, and SLP must know how to ascertain accurate patient responses and how this affects care provision and reimbursement. The skilled disciplines of LPN/LVN, COTA, LPTA, MSS, and dietitian must know how OASIS responses affect the continuum of care they provide over the episode(s). Assessment of OASIS responses should be used to direct care provision and should be used as appropriate to guide the development of the POC.
   New clinical competencies and skills may be required in order to implement best practices that are needed to improve quality of care. Business office managers, data entry, and clerical staff are entering new data and managing agency dollars in different ways.
3. Modify agency processes to support the change in care delivery. Remove obstacles and address inefficiencies. These can include untimely paperwork flow, inefficient work processes, unnecessary documentation requirements, or improperly designed clinical forms that do not meet the clinicians' or patients' needs.

## AGENCY APPLICATION:
### Integrating OASIS Outcomes into Clinical Practice

To what degree has your agency fully integrated OASIS outcomes into clinical practice?

Assess each of the following items and give a brief comment on where your agency is in implementation. Discuss your thoughts among agency leadership.

1. Accurate documentation of patient responses to OASIS items according to CMS response instructions.

_____

_____

_____

_____

2. Accurate OASIS data entry.

_____

_____

_____

_____

3. Transmission of OASIS data according to acceptable time frames.

_____

_____

_____

_____

4. Proper and timely review of OASIS outcome reports.

_____

_____

_____

_____

5. Timely selection of target outcomes for investigation.

_____

_____

_____

_____

**2**B

---

### AGENCY APPLICATION:
### Integrating OASIS Outcomes into Clinical Practice *(continued)*

6. Timely implementation of clinical processes and best practices that should improve outcomes.

_____

_____

_____

_____

7. Demonstrated improvement in outcomes selected for remediation.

_____

_____

_____

_____

---

OASIS and OBQI/OBQM comprise an approach by which patient outcomes can be used to demonstrate home care's effectiveness and quality of care rendered. OASIS provides the vehicle to generate patient outcomes, while OBQI/OBQM provides the tools and criteria to analyze patient outcomes achieved. Performance improvement methods are applied to select and implement changes in care delivery and processes. Successful implementation and use depends upon timely and appropriate outcome report review, selection of target outcomes, application of performance improvement measures to address cause, implementation of best practice standards of care, and formal and informal follow-up.

## REFERENCES

Centers for Medicare and Medicaid Services, U.S. Department of Health and Human Services. (2002). *Outcome-based quality improvement (OBQI) implementation manual.* Baltimore, MD: author.

Crisler, K. S., Baillie, L., & Conway, K. (2003). Using the new OASIS-based reports in OBQI. *Home Healthcare Nurse,* 21(9), 621–626.

Crisler, K. S. & Richard, A. A. (2002a). Developing and implementing a plan of action to improve care: The basics. *Home Healthcare Nurse,* 20(9), 596–602.

Crisler, K. S. & Richard, A. A. (2002b). Interpreting outcome reports: The basics. *Home Healthcare Nurse,* 20(8), 517–522.

Crisler, K. S. & Richard, A. A. (2002c). Selecting target outcomes: The basics. *Home Healthcare Nurse,* 20(8), 525–530.

Crisler, K. S. & Richard, A. A. (2003). New tool to use with patient tally reports. *Home Healthcare Nurse,* 21(9), 627–628.

Department of Health and Human Services, Health Care Financing Administration. (2001). Quality monitoring using case mix and adverse event outcome reports: Implementing outcome-based quality improvement at a home health agency. Retrieved May 30, 2003 from http://www.cms.gov/oasis/obqm1.pdf.

Joint Commission on Accreditation of Healthcare Organizations. (1994). Framework for improving performance: From principles to practice. Oakbrook Terrace, Illinois: author.

Shaugnessy, P. W., Crisler, K. S., Hittle, D. F., & Schlenker, R. E. (2002). Summary of the report on oasis and outcome-based quality improvement in home health care: Research and demonstration findings, policy implications and considerations for future change. Denver, Colorado: Center for Health Services Research, University of Colorado Health Sciences Center.

# Building an Outcome-Based Approach to Home Care

Section C

## Developing Effective, Best Practice Care Pathways

### LEARNING OBJECTIVES

Upon completion of this topic, you will able to:

1. Define care pathway.
2. Describe the purpose of a care pathway.
3. List the components of a care pathway.
4. Develop a care pathway.
5. Prepare for the implementation of care pathways.
6. Aggregate and trend care pathway outcomes data.
7. Analyze and investigate care pathway outcomes data.
8. Integrate clinical pathway outcomes data into clinical practice.

### AGENCY-SPECIFIC DATA/RESOURCES NEEDED

- Current agency care pathway, if used.
- Agency variances from Chapter 1, Section B.

---

**CORE TERMS AND CONCEPTS**

- Care Pathway
- Aggregation & Trending of Pathway Outcomes
- Analyses & Investigation of Pathway Outcomes

*Note: The term care pathway is used generically throughout the remainder of the workbook. It is synonymous with critical pathway, clinical pathway, and the like.*

# INTRODUCTION

Care pathways are not new. They have been used to guide care and measure outcomes, primarily in the acute care setting, for over a decade. However, they have taken on new significance for homecare providers in the wake of prospective pay and outcome-based OASIS. Waggoner (1999) describes them as the "future for homecare agencies."

Knowing how to develop a care pathway is especially useful in providing outcome-based patient care. It gives you the capability to customize care provision for particular referral sources. It enables you to build your standards of care and corresponding outcomes pertinent to the patient populations you serve.

There are many formats for pathways. The format itself is not as critical to achieving outcomes as is the way the standards of care and outcomes are linked within the format. For this reason, this workbook does not endorse a particular format design.

This section guides you through the development of care pathways and the evaluation of existing ones. It also provides recommendations for step-by-step planning, implementation, and follow-up.

## WHAT IS A CARE PATHWAY AND WHAT IS ITS PURPOSE?

A care pathway is *one tool used in the implementation of outcome-based patient care*. It can be described as a blueprint for the clinical management of a diagnosis or condition that outlines a sequence of timed, standard interventions (Humphrey and Malone-Nuzzo, 1996) designed to achieve predictable outcomes (Gingerich and Ondeck, 2000) in a cost-effective way (Waggoner, 1999). Lagoe (1998) states that care pathways are among the most widespread tools used to enhance outcomes and contain costs within a constrained length of stay. Examples of pathways include CHF, COPD, ostomy, pacemaker, pneumonia, asthma, stroke, and dysrhythmia.

Prospective pay means that costs must be actively managed. Managing costs includes managing resources through the number and type of visits made and corresponding interventions. By its design, a care pathway not only provides the avenue to help strategically manage costs, but to project them as well.

The OBQI initiative encourages agencies to incorporate best practices into care delivery for the purposes of remedying or reinforcing patient outcomes (CMS, 2002). Care pathways afford a method by which best practices can be incorporated into scheduled visits. They can also guide clinicians though the measurement of related agency supplemental outcomes in addition to those captured through OASIS.

Because patient and caretaker instruction is central to the delivery of home care, it is prudent to determine how these knowledge outcomes relate to OASIS outcomes that are achieved. Sidorov et al. (2002) found that inadequate knowledge, skills, and motivation about self-care were determinants of adverse health outcomes. Outcomes related to the knowledge and skills necessary for self-care management can be measured by a care pathway and subsequently used to revise standards of care and to improve patient/caretaker teaching materials and methods. These actions have the potential to positively impact the agency's OASIS outcomes as well.

OBQI recommends that agencies determine what the *yardstick* is prior to conducting an outcomes investigation (CMS, 2002). While this critical step is often quite time-consuming and involves review of health care literature and getting a consensus among experienced clinicians, it enables an agency to determine if inappropriate care has been rendered. Investigating OASIS outcomes becomes easier when care pathway interventions are used as the *yardstick* for evaluation of care rendered. Pathway interventions not only guide the care to begin with, but also serve as the *yardstick* for the evaluation of care quality afterwards.

For example, an agency has a less than desired OASIS outcome percentage for *Improvement in pain interfering with activity*. The agency decides to develop a pathway for pain management. The best practices for pain management are included as the interventions on the agency's pathway. These interventions become the *yardstick* by which future outcomes investigations related to pain will be conducted.

## COMPONENTS OF CARE PATHWAYS

The literature (Gingerich and Ondeck, 2001; Fuss and Pasquale, 1998; Hazelip, 2002; Humphrey and Milone-Nuzzo, 1996; Matula, 1995; Strassner, 1997; Waggoner, 1999) reflects these primary components of care pathways:

- Diagnosis, condition or procedure specific
- Interventions specified for each visit, over a planned number of visits
- Cost-effective resource utilization
- Measurement of anticipated outcomes

Other authors (Cole, Houston, and Kite-Powell, 1995; Fuss and Pasquale, 1998; Hill, 1999; Klenner, 2000; Luttman, n.d.; Maturen and Houser (THERF seminar, May 17, 1994); Matula, 1995; Strassner, 1997) include variance as an additional component.

Let's briefly review each component in preparation for developing a care pathway.

**2**c

### 1. Diagnosis, Condition or Procedure Specific

Care pathways are developed for any number of diagnoses, conditions, or procedures. Agencies primarily develop them for high volume, high cost, chronic diagnoses and conditions. These typically reflect diagnoses that are prevalent over a large patient population, such as CHF, diabetes, COPD, and chronic wounds (Smith, 2001). Other care pathways are developed for conditions such as ostomy or pacemaker in an effort to improve continuity of care, to address procedural concerns, and to lower the risks associated with their care.

Large homehealth companies should generate a listing of top diagnoses by volume, and by reimbursement versus cost for each agency, as well as for the company as a whole. This gives each agency director additional perspective for selecting diagnoses for pathway development and management.

### Guiding Questions

- What are the company/agency's top diagnoses by volume? Top conditions?
- Which of these diagnoses are chronic and generally associated with higher treatment costs?
- Which of these diagnoses require the use of problem-prone or high-risk procedures?

### 2. Clinical Interventions

Once you have determined the diagnoses that your staff can best manage via a care pathway, select the clinical interventions. Use clinical practice guidelines, research-based recommendations, clinical expertise, past performance improvement initiatives, and policy and procedure to guide the selection process. *Evaluate each intervention carefully for inclusion in your pathway according to the outcomes you wish to achieve.* Write interventions so that clinicians know specifically **who** is to do **what**, and **when**, facilitating continuity of care among disciplines.

These interventions also form the basis of the care pathway clinical audit for outcome investigations. They should be written so that the reviewer can easily pinpoint issues that may be causing less than desired outcomes.

Determine which of these interventions are necessary for successful patient/caretaker self-management. Give careful consideration to the amount and type of information and skills you deem essential. Prioritize your list, using *have-to-know* versus *nice-to-know* as the basis of your criteria. Also take note of new skill competencies that are required of your staff to implement these interventions.

*Guiding Questions*

- Have we exhausted our search for best practice recommendations?
- Have all essential interventions been included?
- Are there additional interventions that are important for us to consider?
- Will interventions require new or additional staff competency assessments?

### 3. Sequencing of Visits and Clinical Interventions

After the agency formulates the multidisciplinary best practice interventions to implement via the pathway, the painstaking task of assigning a visit or visits to each intervention begins. Examine each intervention closely to determine the skills and amount of information that is essential for patient self-management. For example, the intervention of teaching the disease process of MI may be planned for one visit only, whereas teaching the more complex disease process of diabetes may need to be planned over two-to-three visits.

*Guiding Questions*

- Is there any unnecessary overlap of interventions by disciplines?
- Are too many interventions planned for a single visit?
- Are too many disciplines scheduled for the same day of the week?
- Have we appropriated a sufficient number of visits for teaching patient/caretaker skills, such as injection technique, wound management, infusion, or ostomy management?

### 4. Cost-effective Resource Utilization

A care pathway promotes uniformity and helps to decrease unnecessary use of resources. Attention should be given to the reimbursement for each PPS episode, managed care contract pricing, and the cost of providing care to include salaries, mileage, cost per visit as applicable, and products and supplies. Examine your agency's average visit time for each discipline. Consider your average reimbursement for the diagnosis.

Care pathway design should also include a close evaluation of each discipline's interventions to avoid the duplication of activities and to use the home health aide as effectively as possible. For example, physical and occupational therapists agree that some degree of unnecessary overlap of interventions occurs in certain patient situations. To ensure that this is avoided or kept to a minimum, therapists are encouraged to collaborate and agree to the types of interventions that each will be responsible for. These are reflected in the pathway.

In a second example, a patient is receiving physical therapy and home health aide visits. The therapists determine that aides can provide additional range of motion (ROM). The therapists outline special ROM interventions for the aides. The agency uses these interventions as a standard of care in the pathway.

*Guiding Questions*

- Does visit time need adjustment as a result of selected pathway interventions?
- Is there discipline overlap of interventions?
- Can home health aide visits be used more effectively?
- Does our current average reimbursement for the pathway diagnosis cover the cost of our planned interventions? If not, how can we improve efficiency or cost-effectiveness?

### 5. Measurement of Outcomes

Integrate outcome measurements into existing formats when appropriate. Ensure that outcome indicators are simple, to-the-point, and easy to measure. Remember that agency-written outcomes for pathways are not measured like OASIS outcomes. When using supplemental outcomes, **the agency must decide when each outcome is measured by staff**. The appropriate timeframe must be determined for the first measurement and the end-result measurement, depending upon the subject matter of each outcome. Measurement timeframes for outcomes can vary or they can be the same.

## Guiding Questions

- Is the timeframe for each outcome appropriate? Is it reasonable? Is it possible?
- Is automation feasible?
- If not, what is the most efficient way of measuring outcomes and of obtaining end-result outcomes for use and comparison?

### 6. Variance

After your agency's patient populations have been defined and standards of care and outcomes written, identify the reasons for variance that you will aggregate. Evaluate these closely to ensure that they give perspective to the outcomes that you have chosen to measure via your pathways.

For example, the variances, *difficulty with multiple medications* and *difficulty in reading and writing English,* are appropriate reasons to aggregate because of their effect on outcomes related to patient/caretaker learning in the home setting. *Omission of diagnostic tests* relates to the quality of clinical outcomes achieved and is worthy of aggregation for patients with endocrine disorders, a coagulation deficit, and fluid and electrolyte imbalance.

Decide how to integrate variance data into the care pathway process. Streamline reporting and documenting to optimize staff compliance with this process.

## Guiding Questions

- Will variance data be documented on the pathway? If so, will the pathway be a part of the medical record?
- Does the agency have any objections to its variance data being a part of the medical record?
- If variance is documented outside the medical record, how will the information be reported? How will it be gathered for aggregation?
- Will this process include data entry, individual responsible for PI data, or a senior clinician?

---

### AGENCY APPLICATION:

#### Prioritizing Agency Care Pathways

According to your agency's primary patient population(s), list five care pathways in order of importance that are appropriate for agency implementation.

1. _____

2. _____

3. _____

4. _____

5. _____

---

2c

## CARE PATHWAY DEVELOPMENT VERSUS PURCHASE

Because pathways can be tailored to meet your agency's specific patient population(s), it is helpful for an agency to be able to construct its own care pathways. Agency-developed pathways can also be designed to integrate more smoothly with existing clinical forms or software.

There are many pathways on the market, but proceed with caution and evaluate these carefully prior to purchase. The standards within purchased pathways may or may not contain the interventions needed by an agency to achieve their desired outcomes. Pathways for purchase should be flexible in adding standards and outcomes as necessary.

*Guiding Questions* (for agencies that currently use care pathways)

- Does the agency have pathways for its primary populations?
- Are pathways used consistently and according to agency policy and procedure? If not, specify the reasons.
- Is the pathway format user-friendly? Is it the same for all pathways? Does care pathway documentation duplicate visit note documentation? To what degree? Can this be avoided? Minimized?
- Are agency outcomes aggregated manually or by automation?
- Does the format incorporate standardized patient teaching materials into the interventions?

*Guiding Questions* (when considering purchase)

Does the pathway package:
- Include standards, measurable outcomes, and variance?
- Address at least 10 of the diagnoses and conditions pertinent to my agency's patient population(s)?
- Outline specific interventions for all disciplines or for nursing only?
- Allow for flexibility to add standards, outcomes, or variances as needed?
- Include standardized patient/family teaching materials?
- Integrate well with current clinical forms and agency processes?
- Require manual or automated aggregation of outcomes and variances?
- Include periodic updates?
- Purchase price and implementation costs outweigh its benefits?

## DEVELOPING AN OUTCOME-BASED CARE PATHWAY

Developing care pathways need not be a grueling, time consuming process. There is a methodical way to approach this task. Each step is equally important. The format you select or design should be the same for all pathways used within the agency or company.

### Step 1—Getting started.

Agency leadership staff:
- Support the effort and convey its rationale and importance to all agency staff.
- Consider the resources needed to incorporate care pathways into existing documentation.
- Evaluate the cost of implementation.
- Designate agency representative(s) to participate in pathway development, staff education, and training.
- Approve an implementation action plan and timeline.
- Consider issues related to implementation that may affect weekend and PRN staff.

- Determine when the use of pathways is to begin and how, i.e., with each new admission or conversion of most recent admissions.

*Step 2—Prioritize pathway(s) for development.*

1. Define the agency's primary patient population(s).
2. Identify agency diagnoses or conditions that are appropriate for pathway development.
3. Identify OASIS target outcomes that have potential for improvement through the use of a pathway and the diagnoses/conditions that these outcomes relate to. For example, an agency has a less than desirable OASIS outcome of *Improvement in dyspnea*. It has a large population of CHF patients. A medical record review from patients listed on the OBQI Outcome Tally report reveals interventions are primarily based on individual clinician preference. The agency decides that a care pathway can best meet the needs they have identified.
4. Review average cost and reimbursement pertaining to these diagnoses.
5. Evaluate and identify staff and manager experience and expertise in relation to these diagnoses.

2c

---

## AGENCY APPLICATION:

### Pathway Selection

Name two pathways that you are going to consider for implementation.

1. _____

2. _____

---

*Step 3—Develop a format that will be used for all care pathways.*

Explore different formats for designing your care pathway. Any format that is efficient, user-friendly, integrates well with current agency documentation, and contains the necessary components is acceptable. Select categories of care that encompass all multidisciplinary clinical interventions you will use. This helps ensure the pathways are uniform for all diagnoses and conditions. Following are several categories with example interventions ("Critical Pathways—An Acute," 1994; Klenner, 2000; Maturen and Houser, 1994) (An agency may use any number of categories or rename categories as it feels appropriate):

- *Assessment(s)* (includes physical, pressure ulcer risk, fall risk, pain, home safety)
- *Diagnostic tests* (lab, EKG, pulse oximetry)
- *Procedures* (performed by staff) (irrigations, infusion therapy)
- *Disease Process* (pathophysiology/recognition and reporting of adverse signs and symptoms)
- *Medications* (actions, side effects, dosage, precautions, interactions)
- *Nutrition/Hydration* (special diet, fluid requirements and restrictions, and dietary guidelines, such as those recommended for wound healing, increased need of iron-rich foods, increased fiber)
- *Mobility/Rehabilitation* (turning, active/passive ROM, home exercise program, resistance training, strengthening, flexibility, and balance)
- *Safety/Equipment Management* (adjustments to environment, proper use and cleaning of equipment)

- *Psychosocial* (temporary or permanent adjustments to lifestyle, work, recreation)
- *Pain Management* (methods of pain control)
- *Self-Management Skills* (includes skills that must be acquired by the patient or care-taker to properly manage the condition in the absence of the healthcare provider. For example, wound dressing removal/cleansing and re-application, use of glucometer, foot care, infant CPR, managing an infusion, use of food journal.)

**Step 4—Determine if best practices have been recommended for these two diagnoses/conditions.**

- Access websites. (See Appendix A: Internet Resource Listing: Best Practices.) Review the published health literature.
- Determine if your agency has established additional standards of care through performance improvement initiatives. Incorporate these standards as needed.

*Suggestion:*

Have agency Admin/Nursing Director meet with agency's medical director or high volume referral source related to the two pathway Dxs or conditions. Allow for feedback regarding outlined pathway interventions and outcomes. Consider other customers' recommendations, if any.

---

### AGENCY APPLICATION:
#### Identifying Resources

1. Identify the individual(s) who will research the literature or websites.

   _____

   _____

2. Identify the potential source(s) of information for best practice.

   _____

   _____

3. Conduct your search.

---

**Step 5—List published best practice recommendations for these two pathways.**

- Outline *best practices* that you will evaluate for pathway interventions.

---

### AGENCY APPLICATION:
#### Selecting Best Practices

1. Use the *Best Practices Research Tool* (Appendix E1) to record your findings.
2. Use care pathway categories to organize best practice interventions.
3. Make additional copies of the worksheet as needed.

*Step 6—Conduct medical record reviews.*

Select a random sample of agency's patients who have been admitted with one of the two selected primary diagnoses over the last 12 months. (See page 124–125.)

- Outline practice patterns of physicians with high-volume referrals. *Important:* Note any routine physician orders that identify a standard of care or outcomes expectations for incorporation into pathways. Homecare providers may overlook this valuable source of information.
  For example, an orthopedic surgeon has routine orders that include discharging the patient when a certain degree of independence is achieved. This directive can be converted into a measurable outcome indicator to be used by staff, such as *Patient is able to transfer independently from bed to wheelchair prior to discharge.*
- Note patient teaching materials and methods used. Note presence or lack of standardization. Does the agency direct the use of standard teaching materials for certain topics or does the clinician select materials of his or her choice?
- Note interventions for all disciplines.
- Compile information from chart review findings for baseline data and comparison. Also note average number of visits per diagnosis per episode by discipline. Note average reimbursement per diagnosis per episode and average cost per diagnosis per episode.

2c

---

### AGENCY APPLICATION:
### Conducting Medical Record Review

1. Use the *Chart Audit Tool: Current Agency Practice* (Appendix E2) to record interventions found in your medical record review. Make additional copies as needed.
2. Identify who will participate in medical record review.

_____

_____

3. Identify physicians who have standing or routine orders for either of your two selected diagnoses/conditions. Closely examine these orders for outcomes.
4. Note orders that are reflective of best practice recommendations and are appropriate for inclusion in the pathways.
5. According to record review findings, list the interventions, including teaching material and resources, that are currently being provided by each discipline for these diagnoses.
6. Use the care pathway categories on the audit tool to organize interventions.

---

*Step 7—Compare published best practices with current agency practice.*

- Compare and contrast best practice recommendations with your agency's current practice.
  *Note: You also may have a current agency intervention that is policy, even though you may not find it in published best practice.*
- Re-evaluate the policy in light of best practice and include it in the pathway, as you deem appropriate.

---

## AGENCY APPLICATION:

### Selecting Interventions for Your Agency Care Pathway

1. Use the *Best Practices/Interventions by Discipline Worksheet* (Appendix E3) to record your selected interventions. Use additional copies as needed.
2. Compare and contrast the interventions you entered for best practice in *Step 5* with interventions from chart review in *Step 6*.
3. Highlight the interventions from steps five and six that are applicable and appropriate for your agency's primary patient populations and goals, according to the discipline you feel most qualified to perform the intervention.
4. Enter the highlighted interventions by discipline on the *Worksheet* (Appendix E3).

---

*Step 8—Closely examine the interventions you outlined for each discipline.*

Do any overlap across disciplines? For example, look at the provisions of exercise, safety instruction, adaptation of home environment for care.

Does any overlap exist here? If so, specify.

_____

_____

_____

_____

_____

Determine which discipline is most appropriate to provide this care and during which visit. Re-adjust pathway as needed.

*Step 9—Determine the number of visits per discipline that will be needed to provide each pathway intervention.*

- Review the agency's **current** average number of visits per discipline for the pathway diagnoses/conditions.
- Look at the pathway interventions you assigned to each discipline.
- Assign the number of visits needed to implement each intervention and to help achieve desired outcomes.
- Evaluate the need for adjusting average visit times to accommodate interventions.
  *Note: Financial considerations for pathway development are discussed in Chapter 4.*

## AGENCY APPLICATION:

### Planning Specific Visit Interventions

Use the *Pathway Intervention and Episode Planning Tool* (Appendix E4) for this application.

1. Use the key at top of form. Copy this form for the number of weeks/episodes needed. Note the following example in Table 2.1 for the patient with multiple sclerosis.
2. Enter the total number of visits planned for <u>each</u> intervention. Patient is admitted on Wednesday. The letter "P" is placed in each box that corresponds to visits that PT plans to make; an "N" for those Nursing plans to make.
3. Enter the total # of disciplines per day and visits per week at the bottom of the page.

**TABLE 2.1** Pathway Interventions and Episode Planning Tool

| Pathway: Multiple Sclerosis | Wk #1 | | | | | | | | Wk #2 | | | | | | | |
|---|---|---|---|---|---|---|---|---|---|---|---|---|---|---|---|---|
| Enter agency's Medicare weekdays | M | T | W | Th | F | Sa | Su | | M | T | W | Th | F | Sa | Su |
| *Interventions* | *Planned Visits* | | | | | | | | | | | | | | |
| **Medications** | 6 | | | N | | N | | | | | N | | N | | |
| **Mobility/Rehabilitation** | | | | | | | | | | | | | | | |
| 1. Exercise program | 14 | | | P | | P | | | | P | | P | | P | |
| **# of Disciplines per Day** | | | | 2 | | 2 | | | | 1 | 1 | 1 | | 2 | |
| **Total Visits: per Week / per Episode** | 4 | / | — | | | | | | 5 | / | — | | | | |

### Guiding Questions

- Does the pathway need further adjustment to be more efficient and cost-effective, without adversely affecting quality of care?
- Have visits been planned for each discipline as appropriate?
- What rationale is used to determine number of visits and interventions provided during the visits?

*Step 10—Evaluate your agency's current patient teaching materials relative to best practices for selected diagnoses.*

- Determine if new or revised materials are needed for patient/family use.
- Decide if material is available for purchase or if material can be written from within. If developed from within, designate individual(s) responsible for this task.
- Organize patient teaching material file or library for easy staff access.

*Guiding Questions*

- Does patient teaching material reflect best practices?

---

## AGENCY APPLICATION:

### Selecting Information for Patient Teaching Materials

Use the *Teaching Material Worksheet* (Appendix E5) for this application.

1. Specify the topics and corresponding information that will be included in the agency's standardized patient teaching material based on the interventions that are implemented.
2. Enter topics and related information on *Worksheet*. Make additional copies as needed.

---

**Step 11—***Determine if any additions or changes to product lines or supplies will be needed to enhance implementation of these pathways.*

- Identify and evaluate the supplies/products/product lines.
- Agency leadership staff to make recommendations.

---

## AGENCY APPLICATION:

### Evaluating Product Lines and Supplies

Specify the supplies/product lines that are needed, if any, and state your rationale.

_____

_____

_____

_____

_____

---

**Step 12—***Identify supplemental outcome indicators that will be measured for the two diagnoses/conditions.*

- Establish a set of outcomes that each pathway will measure and that coincide directly with the standards of care you have chosen to implement.
- Design a format that allows the clinician to measure each outcome within established agency time frames. The clinician must document if the patient met or did not meet the outcome, and if the outcome was not applicable to the patient. Each outcome should be listed and noted by a clinician's checkmark, date, or other notation that indicates the outcome measurement made by the clinician.
- If your agency chooses to use an established valid and reliable clinical outcome measurement scale, such as NOC, compare your outcome needs to those listed within the scale. Make sure the outcome measurements capture outcomes relative to your agency's best practice interventions.

- Look at each category in the pathway, and then note the standards within each that you have decided to implement. *Determine the outcome that you want to achieve by providing that particular intervention.* For example, an ADA standard of care for the diabetic patient is teaching the recognition and management of hypo/hyperglycemia by (agency timeframe). An appropriate outcome that corresponds to this teaching intervention is *Patient/caretaker verbalizes signs/symptoms of hypo/hyperglycemia.*

  *Note: It is important to remember that an outcome does not have to be measured for every intervention.* However, you must evaluate each intervention to decide which corresponding outcomes are pertinent for measurement. Evaluate each pathway intervention relative to the outcome you wish to achieve until all interventions have been evaluated. Then determine the number of outcome indicators you wish to measure by prioritizing them according to quality of care issues, risks, volume, agency goals, or other concerns or interest.

---

### AGENCY APPLICATION:

### Writing Pathway Outcome Indicators

Use the *Supplemental Outcome Indicator Worksheet* (Appendix E6) for this application.

1. Evaluate each pathway intervention to determine if a desired outcome measurement is warranted. If so, write the outcome in measurable terms on the *Worksheet*. Include the discipline(s) that measure the outcome and the timeframe in which it is measured. Use additional copies as needed.
2. When you are finished writing the first pathway's outcomes, re-evaluate them to determine if an important outcome was overlooked or if an unnecessary outcome was written.

---

*Step 13—Determine if additional staff competencies are required for pathway best practice interventions.*

- Identify those competencies required per discipline for each diagnosis.
- Decide which competencies require demonstration or written testing.
- Designate individual(s) to design competency assessments as needed, and to provide competency training and education, as necessary.

2c

## AGENCY APPLICATION:

### Selecting Pathway Competencies

List competencies needing testing or review and how each will be assessed:

Pathway 1: _____    Pathway 2: _____

SN _____    _____

_____    _____

_____    _____

THERAPY _____    _____

_____    _____

_____    _____

HHA _____    _____

_____    _____

_____    _____

Specify who will be conducting competency assessments for each discipline:

_____

_____

_____

_____

_____

_____

_____

_____

_____

*Step 14—Identify pathway variances that the agency will track.*

Determine how pathway variances will be reported or documented.

*Guiding Questions*

- Will these variances be documented in the permanent record or aside from visit note or pathway documentation?
- How will variances be extrapolated from the documentation? Will this occur during daily data entry?
- How will variances be aggregated, manually, or via automation?

---

### AGENCY APPLICATION:

#### Selecting Variances

In addition to the agency variances you chose in Chapter 1, Section B, are there others your agency wants to report and aggregate? If so, list these below.

_____

_____

_____

---

## PREPARING FOR PATHWAY IMPLEMENTATION

**2**c

*Step 1—Evaluate existing clinical documentation format.*

- Evaluate your pathway format, manual or automated, in relation to clinical forms or screens that are currently in use.
- Look specifically for overlap in documentation requirements of staff. Avoid this if at all possible. Duplicate documentation adversely affects staff efficiency and compliance and can impede use or prevent success.

*Guiding Questions*

- If there is overlap or duplication, is there any possible way to avoid it?
- Are there documentation adjuncts to the clinical note currently in use, such as flow sheets, that will continue as an adjunct to the use of a pathway?
- Can staff document the interventions on the pathway itself, making it a part of the medical record?
- If manual, where will the pathway be located for easy access?

*Step 2—Consider the use of automation to improve efficiency.*

- Evaluate existing agency software applications to determine if these can provide automation of part or all of the pathway documents. For example, can manual documentation of the pathway be entered by data entry staff on a daily basis to keep pathway documentation current for the next clinician's visit?
- Evaluate point-of-care devices.
- Evaluate scanning technology.

*Step 3—Evaluate existing automation to enhance efficiency.*

Automation does not always guarantee efficiency. If it takes more than one hour to document the admission of a patient on a pathway, an evaluation of the pathway design or format is in order.

*Guiding Questions*

- Do staff have to scroll or page down through multiple screens to access pathway interventions and outcomes?
- Does the link between standards and outcomes need to be improved by delineating specifically what the agency requires?

*Step 4—Determine the process that staff will use to initiate the use of a pathway.*

Clinicians may not know which pathway to initiate until the admission assessment is completed. In this case, it may be necessary to initiate the pathway on visit two. Include this in policy.

### Guiding Questions

*On admission:*
- How will staff access the pathway?
- How is it going to be initiated?
- Will only one pathway be initiated on admission?

*When the diagnosis changes during an episode:*
- How is the pathway accessed?
- Will the patient continue on the pathway initiated on admission and add an additional (second pathway) if the primary diagnosis changes mid-episode?

*Step 5—Evaluate how patient teaching material is to be organized and accessed by clinicians.*

Patient teaching material must be organized for efficiency and must be available at all times, including weekends and evenings.

### Guiding Questions

- Does the pathway direct the use of specific teaching materials relative to the standard interventions?
- Where are the patient teaching materials located? Office library, filing cabinet?
- How are patient teaching materials organized? Alphabetically according to diagnosis? Will materials be located with their manual pathway counterparts?

*Step 6—Provide pathway instructions for use to clinical staff. Consider the following topics:*

- Introduction to outcome-based practice/How outcomes are used
- The crucial role of the clinician in measuring outcomes
- Differences in pathways vs. usual care
- Standards of Care/Best Practices
- Patient/Family teaching materials as a standard
- How to measure outcomes
- Reporting/documenting variance and timeliness of variance documentation
- Importance of accurate outcomes measurement
- Integration of pathways into practice

## PATHWAY IMPLEMENTATION AND FOLLOW-UP

## Implementation

The success of pathway implementation can be dependent upon the number of pathways concurrently implemented. Leadership commitment to managing the change plays a key role in success. If you decide to implement only one initially, you should select a pathway of high volume to allow staff to become accustomed to the new process in a more timely manner.

Educate all staff that are affected by care pathways to the details of the processes that your agency will implement. For example, home health aides are likely to play an important role in your agency's management of a pressure ulcer. Classes may include teaching them how to properly identify and report patient risk for development of an ulcer or a stage I ulcer, to report poor food intake, to apply proper pressure reduction, and to properly use a turning schedule. Inform them of how these actions on their aide assignment support those on the pathway for the SN and therapists, as applicable.

### Guiding Questions

- Have we considered how the process will work during the evenings and on weekends?
- Have we recognized any obstacles in the process that have not been addressed?

## Implementation Follow-Up

### Formal

- Conduct follow-up three-to-four weeks into implementation.
- Conduct medical record reviews to evaluate implementation of interventions against pathway standards.
- Obtain feedback from staff meetings or surveys. Share composite with staff.
- Ask for suggestions when you make revisions to the process or to forms.

### Informal

All agency managers and those involved in the development process should take every opportunity to spend a few moments in one-on-one discussions with staff to encourage, educate, clarify directives, evaluate compliance, correct misunderstood procedure, obtain feedback on the process, and identify obstacles that arise. Many times managers wait to discuss issues in formal staff meetings or in educational sessions that typically get cancelled or rescheduled. Taking advantage of these brief encounters also lets your staff know that successful implementation of the process is important to you.

## AGGREGATION AND TRENDING OF CARE PATHWAY OUTCOMES DATA

Because the aggregation and trending of outcomes data is a powerful tool in patient management, marketing, finance management, and PI, agency leadership should understand how to perform these calculations for agency supplemental outcomes.

To aggregate outcomes is to *generate a total* (Merriam-Webster, 2002) *percent or average of patients (having the same diagnosis or like conditions):*

- who have met or achieved each outcome (Klenner, 2000)
- who have not met or not achieved each outcome (Klenner, 2000)
- for whom each outcome is not applicable (J. W. Anderton, personal communication, April 15, 1991)

The aggregate is expressed as a proportion or ratio that shows the number of occurrences compared to the entire group within which the occurrence could take place (Joint Commission, 1994). For example, you have 100 patients for whom an outcome is measured. Eighty patients *Met* or achieved the outcome. The aggregate for this outcome is expressed as:

$$\frac{80 \text{ patients who met the outcome}}{100 \text{ total patients for whom the outcome applies}} = 80\% \text{ Met or achieved the outcome}$$

Using aggregated information from pathways is similar to using OASIS outcome reports; they both give agency results or outcomes in percentages for the population of patients having the outcome(s) measured. Desirable outcomes achieved and those that need remediation can then be noted.

Data is aggregated at a frequency appropriate to the activity or process being studied (Joint Commission, 2004) or measured. For example, an outcome that is measured for a small number of patients may require an aggregation over 12 months to have enough data to draw meaningful conclusions.

*Aggregation* can be performed manually or through software application. While automation is more efficient, you should understand how to perform the calculations manually. Then you can express these needs to information systems (IS) in the event you choose to automate your agency's supplemental outcomes data.

*Trending* of outcomes data is critical to performance improvement efforts. It allows for periodic comparing of one's own data over time and also with external benchmarks when available (Joint Commission, 2004). Outcomes data are transposed from the format for aggregation to a format for trending that shows aggregates for each quarter or month in the year, or results from year to year. This allows you to note excessive variability (Joint Commission, 2004) and to determine if outcomes (results) are improving, worsening, or remaining the same over time.

You should trend data month-to-month or quarter-to-quarter. Large agencies may find the volume of data easier to manage when aggregated month-to-month. A bar graph is an excellent method of depicting trends.

---

## CONCEPT APPLICATION (1):

### Aggregating Supplemental Outcome Percentages

An agency is ready to aggregate care pathway outcome measures for all patients who have been admitted with a primary diagnosis of pressure ulcer in the last quarter. The following is a sample of the agency's outcomes that are measured via a pressure ulcer pathway:

1. Patient/caretaker verbalizes S/S of wound deterioration and infection by visit five.
2. Patient/caretaker verbalizes sources of protein and calories in the diet and states how these nutrients affect healing by visit four.
3. Patient/caretaker verbalizes how to use the proper timeframe for turning by visit two.
4. Patient/caretaker demonstrates methods to obtain pressure relief by visit four.
5. Patient/caretaker demonstrates how to properly change the wound dressing by visit seven.

*Step 1*

Count the total number of patients in the group for whom the outcomes were measured.

*Example:* An agency had 20 patients with pressure ulcers in the last quarter for whom outcomes were measured.  N = 20.

*Step 2*

For each outcome, total the number of patients in this group:

- Who met or achieved the outcome
- Who did not meet or achieve the outcome
- Who did not have the outcome apply to them

## CONCEPT APPLICATION (1):

### Aggregating Supplemental Outcome Percentages *(continued)*

In this concept application, five pressure ulcer outcomes are aggregated.

| Outcomes | # Met / # Applicable = % Met | # Not Met / # Applicable = % Not Met | # NA / # N = % NA |
|---|---|---|---|
| 1 | 20 / 20 = 100% | 0 / 20 = 0% | 0 / 20 = 0% |
| 2 | 19 / 19 = 100% | 0 / 19 = 0% | 1 / 20 = 5% |
| 3 | 20 / 20 = 100% | 0 / 20 = 0% | 0 / 20 = 0% |
| 4 | 15 / 20 = 75% | 5 / 20 = 25% | 0 / 20 = 0% |
| 5 | 12 / 17 = 70% | 5 / 17 = 29% | 3 / 20 = 15% |

*Note: The # Applicable (number of patients for whom the outcome is applicable) is the same number used in the calculation of both met and not met outcome percentages. (# Met + # Not Met = # Applicable)*

For outcome indicator #1 (patient/caretaker verbalizes S/S of wound deterioration/infection) all 20 patients met or achieved the outcome. Determine the percentage of total patients meeting the outcome by setting up a simple proportion:

Twenty patients met the outcome (divided by) 20 patients for whom the outcome applied equals 100% of the patients who met the outcome in this patient group. 20 / 20 = 100%

For outcome indicator #5 (patient/caretaker demonstrates how to properly change the wound dressing) 12 patients met the outcome, 5 patients did not meet the outcome, and 3 patients/caretakers had wound dressings changed by the homecare clinician. Simple percentages are calculated for this patient group who met and who did not meet the outcome, as well as the percentage of all patients for whom the outcome did not apply.

- Twelve patients met the outcome (divided by) 17 patients for whom the outcome applied (equals) 70% of this patient group who met or achieved the outcome. 12 / 17 = 70%
- Five patients did not meet the outcome (divided by) 17 patients for whom the outcome applied (equals) 29% of this patient group who did not meet the outcome. 5 / 17 = 29%
- The outcome did not apply to three patients. Three patients (divided by) 20 total patients (equals) 15% of this group for whom the outcome did not apply. 3 / 20 = 15%

2c

## AGENCY APPLICATION (1):

### Aggregating Supplemental Outcome Percentages

Aggregate the following outcomes. Enter the percentage of patients who met each outcome, who did not meet each outcome, and the percentage of patients for whom the outcome did not apply.  Total number (N) of discharged patients is 15. Refer to the Outcomes Aggregation Summary (Appendix E7) for future agency use.

| Outcomes | # Met / # Applicable = % Met | # Not Met / # Applicable = % Not Met | # NA / # N = % NA |
|---|---|---|---|
| 1 | 13 / 15 = _____ | 2 / 15 = _____ | 0 / _____ = _____ |
| 2 | 14 / 14 = _____ | 0 / 14 = _____ | 1 / _____ = _____ |
| 3 | 15 / 15 = _____ | 0 / 15 = _____ | 0 / _____ = _____ |
| 4 | 12 / 15 = _____ | 3 / 15 = _____ | 0 / _____ = _____ |
| 5 | 11 / 13 = _____ | 2 / 13 = _____ | 2 / _____ = _____ |

### Guiding Questions

- Is every percentage or a vast majority 100%? If so, are these results unlikely for the type of patients you are aggregating? If so, are these results likely or unlikely for the number of patients you are aggregating?
- If calculations are manual, is the math correct?
- Are outcomes measured accurately?
- Does documentation in the record(s) correlate with outcomes achieved?

*Answers:*

| Outcomes | # Met / # Applicable = % Met | # Not Met / # Applicable = % Not Met | # NA / # N = % NA |
|---|---|---|---|
| 1 | 13 / 15 =  86% | 2 / 15 = 13% | 0 / 15 =  0% |
| 2 | 14 / 14 = 100% | 0 / 14 =  0% | 1 / 15 =  6% |
| 3 | 15 / 15 = 100% | 0 / 15 =  0% | 0 / 15 =  0% |
| 4 | 12 / 15 =  80% | 3 / 15 = 20% | 0 / 15 =  0% |
| 5 | 11 / 13 =  84% | 2 / 13 = 15% | 2 / 15 = 13% |

## CONCEPT APPLICATION (2):

### Trending Outcome Percentages

The agency has aggregated outcomes data for two consecutive quarters. Let's trend the data that we aggregated for the five outcomes for the 20 pressure ulcer patients in Concept Application (1).

**Agency Trending Report**

| Outcomes | 1stQ | 2ndQ | 1stQ | 2ndQ | 1stQ | 2ndQ |
|---|---|---|---|---|---|---|
| | % MET | | % NOT MET | | % NA | |
| 1) Verbalizes S/S wound deterioration/infection | 100 | 88 | 0 | 12 | 0 | 0 |
| 2) Verbalizes protein/ calorie needs | 100 | 100 | 0 | 0 | 5 | 0 |
| 3) Verbalizes Q 2hr turning schedule | 100 | 100 | 0 | 0 | 0 | 0 |
| 4) Demonstrates pressure relief | 75 | 100 | 15 | 0 | 0 | 0 |
| 5) Demonstrates dressing of wound | 70 | 75 | 29 | 25 | 15 | 0 |

In this example, for the first quarter, 100% of 20 patients with pressure ulcers *Met* outcome #1, *verbalizes s/s wound deterioration/infection*. However, in the second quarter, only 88% of the patients with pressure ulcers were able to *verbalize s/s of wound deterioration/infection.*

In the agency's initial overview of this outcome, the total number of pressure ulcer patients was smaller in the second quarter; this could contribute to this drop in percentage. However, these records were reviewed to reveal that caretakers of these particular patients were elderly and had difficulty with recall.

Notice outcome #5 above. Agency trending reveals improvement. In the first quarter, only 70% of the patient/caretakers with pressure ulcers were able to *demonstrate proper dressing of the wound*. The agency targeted this outcome and implemented a PI initiative to improve it.

This initiative positively impacted this outcome, as shown by *trending the outcomes data* for both the first and second quarters of the year. However, the agency is not satisfied with 75% and wants to achieve further improvement in the outcome. In a brainstorming session, staff make specific recommendations to further enhance care and to conduct another follow-up chart review. Variances for this population were also reviewed in relation to these outcomes data to see how they impacted the outcome percentages. A sizeable percentage of patients who had difficulty dressing the wound had difficulty reading and writing and had frequent change in caretakers.

2c

## AGENCY APPLICATION (2):

### Trending Outcome Percentages

Transpose the outcome percentages you aggregated in Agency Application (1) to the 3rd Quarter of the Trending Report below.

**Agency Trending Report**

| Outcomes | 1stQ | 2ndQ | 3rdQ | | 1stQ | 2ndQ | 3rdQ | | 1stQ | 2ndQ | 3rdQ | |
|---|---|---|---|---|---|---|---|---|---|---|---|---|
| | | % MET | | | | % NOT MET | | | | % NA | | |
| 1) | 100 | 88 | ( | ) | 0 | 12 | ( | ) | 0 | 0 | ( | ) |
| 2) | 100 | 100 | ( | ) | 0 | 0 | ( | ) | 5 | 0 | ( | ) |
| 3) | 100 | 100 | ( | ) | 0 | 0 | ( | ) | 0 | 0 | ( | ) |
| 4) | 75 | 100 | ( | ) | 15 | 0 | ( | ) | 0 | 0 | ( | ) |
| 5) | 70 | 75 | ( | ) | 29 | 25 | ( | ) | 15 | 0 | ( | ) |

### Guiding Questions

- Which outcome percentages have positive trends?
- Which outcome percentages have negative trends?
- Which outcome percentages have remained the same?
- What are agency variances that may have affected trends?
- Are there wide swings in percentages for the same outcome? If so, is this due to a greater variability in patient numbers?

## ANALYSIS AND INVESTIGATION OF CARE PATHWAY OUTCOMES DATA

Even though outcomes can be measured, aggregated, interpreted, and analyzed in a variety of ways, PI essentially drives the subsequent investigation of outcomes data. Analysis and investigation should be conducted not less than quarterly.

*Note: While the steps below are outlined sequentially, they can be undertaken simultaneously.*

### Step 1—Designate a member of leadership to facilitate outcomes evaluation and interpretation.

Involve the agency's leadership team and clinical staff throughout the process.

### Step 2—Evaluate outcome percentages for patterns that indicate a red flag.

For example, are all of the percentages or the vast majority of all calculated as 100% met? If so, staff may not be measuring the outcomes accurately. Are they using appropriate agency definitions when measuring the outcomes? This can be addressed through staff meetings and discussion, staff development, and/or staff accountability.

*Step 3—Verify the accuracy of your outcomes data.*

Are staff measuring outcomes according to definition? And at the appropriate time? If outcomes aggregation is automated, are outcomes entered accurately into the computer system?

*Step 4—Perform manual calculations for outcome percentages, if necessary.*

If calculations are done manually, check for accuracy.
Review Met, Not Met, and Not Applicable percentages for each outcome for all pathways.

*Step 5—Conduct an overview of all outcomes achieved.*

*Step 6—Prioritize and select outcomes needing further investigation.*

Set initial thresholds for acceptable outcome percentages achieved.
*\*Note: A threshold may be established by the agency over a period of time while initially collecting data. Thresholds should be flexible, increasing as outcomes improve. Thresholds may also be established by reviewing the health literature and research. For example, if compliance with diet and medications is 50% nationally for CHF patients, a threshold of 65–75% may be a worthwhile threshold to set **initially** for CHF outcomes related to diet and medication.*

2c

- Review all outcomes percentages for each pathway.
- Highlight percentages that are below expectations or agency established thresholds.
- Focus on the outcome(s) of a diagnosis, condition, or procedure that:
  1. has quality of care as a potential issue.
  2. is high cost to treat in relation to reimbursement.
  3. is typically high volume.
  4. is problematic in some way.
  5. is of major concern for another reason.
- Target outcomes for investigation that have the greatest impact on quality of care rendered, financial management, or strategic plan and/or choose an unacceptable outcome percentage that is common to multiple diagnoses or conditions. For example, the outcome *patient/family verbalizes dose, action, three main side effects, precautions and food/drug interactions of all medications* has an unacceptably low percentage for several diagnoses and conditions.
  *\*Note: Significance, which is reported for OASIS outcomes, is not typically reported for agency care pathways*

*Step 7—Review demographics specifically for your patient population during the same time period that care is provided to give perspective to your outcome percentages.*

Outcome reports for care pathways are typically generated according to diagnosis or condition and patient demographics. An agency may want to consider having IS develop a link between the agency's existing patient demographics software and the agency's outcomes data. Patient demographics data are entered into the agency's software system on admission. At least on a quarterly basis, the agency aggregates its outcomes data according to a diagnosis and specific demographic data of its choice.

For example, the agency's aggregation of outcomes for patients with a fractured hip is automated via agency software. The agency's software system has been designed to filter any number of demographics or patient characteristics according to choice:

Time period of review
Primary Diagnosis: Fractured Hip
Co-Morbid conditions (Secondary Dxs)

Age group
Lives alone
Physician
Patient Locale
Payer Source
Other: As programmed by choice into the agency's computer database.
*Note: Also review OASIS Case Mix Profile Report information.*

**Step 8—Determine the likely cause of the outcome(s) needing remediation or reinforcement.**

- Brainstorm with clinical staff.
- Form a focus group or PI team as appropriate to initiate PI efforts.
- Identify the approach(es) that will be used to investigate care (Staff Interviews/ Discussions/Questionnaire, Review of staff competency, Home Visit Observation, and Medical record review).

*Note: Because best practice interventions are designed to achieve specific outcomes, the outcomes investigation will focus primarily on whether these best practice interventions or standards of care were implemented according to management expectations.*

## Guiding Questions

- Do staff properly implement the standard?
- Do staff run into obstacles as they implement standards of care?
- Do staff know the standards and when to implement them?
- Does one or more of the standards need revision?
- Review the agency's current patient education materials specific to the diagnosis, condition, or procedure. Has the agency adopted a specific set of "standard" education materials to use? Do staff select materials of their choice?
- Are staff compliant with using standard teaching materials?
- Are there obstacles to staff obtaining these materials?
- Are patient teaching materials clear enough, legible, simply written, and available in other languages as needed?
- What method is used when the patient/caretaker cannot read or knows little English?

*Concerning medical record review*
- Who will facilitate this activity? Include clinical staff in this review.
- Does a special chart audit tool need to be designed to review care? To tally results? Who will devise these tools?
- Formulate your clinical chart audit tool to incorporate your standard(s) of care. Keep the audit tool simple. Focus on the standards.
- Who will review care rendered?

*Note: Medical record review is a critical component of investigating patient outcomes data. Proper selection of a random sample of patients for this review is equally important.*

*Selecting a systematic random sample (Polit, Beck, and Hungler, 2001)*

1. *Define the population:* For example, all patients with a primary diagnosis of pressure ulcer discharged in the 2nd Quarter of 2004.
2. *Determine sample size.* Sample size needs to represent characteristics of the population size. For example, if only 10 patients had a primary diagnosis of pressure ulcer, it is prudent to use all 10 patients in your sample. If 75 patients had the primary diagnosis of pressure ulcer, your sample should be larger. A sample size of 15

to 20 patients would be more appropriate. The larger the sample size, the more representative of the population being investigated.

3. *Select a random sample of patient records to be reviewed from the population that has been identified.* For example, generate a list of all patients with a primary diagnosis of pressure ulcer discharged between the dates of April 1, 2004 and June 30, 2004.
   - Choose the first patient on the list by chance.
   - Choose every patient thereafter according to a sampling interval, which is the standard distance between selected elements. For example, the patient list contains **60 patients** with primary diagnosis of CHF. You select your **sample size** to be **15**. The sampling interval is **(60/15 = 4)**.
   - Select the first name by chance and then every 4th name thereafter until you have 15 records for review. Thus, if your first patient name selected by chance was 10th on the list, the next name in your sample would be 14th; the next name would be 18th and so on.

### Step 9—Aggregate and summarize findings.

List the aspects of care found during staff interviews, chart reviews, home visit observation, financial reviews, and other documentation that seemed to be problematic and that have the greatest potential for improving unacceptable care pathway outcome(s).

Now state these or display these in specific detail. You can apply graphs, charts, or other PI methods to display investigation results and to prioritize those you will address.

For example:
- Only 45% of weekend SN staff can verbalize the process for initiating a care pathway on admission.
- The agency's standardized teaching material for myocardial infarction is distributed to only 70% of the patients having MI as their admitting diagnosis.
- The agency does not use a specific fall risk assessment tool.
- Agency costs exceed reimbursement for the treatment of pressure ulcers 38% of the time by at least $232.00 per episode.

Review aggregated variances for same report period under review.

### Step 10—Select specifics of care delivery that need to be changed to improve outcomes or those that need to be reinforced to maintain desired outcomes.

For example, is it an improved assessment? Specific interventions? Better care planning? Policy and procedure? Improved communication? Better evaluation? Improved staff accountability? Process issues?

### Step 11—Develop a plan of action.

- Appoint an individual to facilitate writing the plan. Keep it simple.
- Appoint clinically qualified individuals to review best practice recommendations and to review and revise standards of care as needed.
- Determine what resources, if any, are needed to implement these best practice recommendations.
- Determine how to procure these resources.
- Outline components of staff education required to implement best practices. Will staff need new or additional skills and related competency assessments? When will this training take place? Who will provide training? Where will training take place? On-site, off-site?
- Include best practice standards and respective skills in new employee orientation.
- Determine how and when all remaining staff will be informed of these findings and of the implementation date of the new or revised standards.

*Step 12—Implement best practices.*

As appropriate, discuss a best practices or a standard of care with the agency Medical Director.

*\*Note: When an agency adopts a particular standard of care, the patient's physician must approve the intervention for it to become a part of the patient's plan of care.*

*Step 13—Perform implementation follow-up.*

- Perform follow-up within four weeks of implementation.
- Get feedback from management and clinical staff.
- Conduct a follow-up medical record review as necessary.
- Perform aggregation of agency outcomes data and variances. Determine if percentages are acceptable for your agency.
- Review trending or begin trending of outcomes data.
- Provide detailed follow-up feedback to all management and clinical staff.
- Reinforce acceptable outcomes achieved and continue to investigate and improve those that are unacceptable.
  *\*Note: This is the cycle that forms the basis of continuous PI.*
- Celebrate successes.

---

## AGENCY APPLICATION:

### Improving OASIS Outcomes through a Care Pathway

- Review your agency's OASIS Risk-Adjusted and Descriptive Outcomes Report for a select time period.
- Review your agency's OASIS Case Mix Profile Report for the same time period.
- Using the concepts and application practice that you have gained thus far, select one OASIS target outcome(s) for investigation.
- Determine if any of your agency's top diagnoses relate to the outcome(s) you have targeted.
- Complete your agency's investigation of the target outcome(s).
- Determine if a care pathway is a suitable method to improve the target outcome(s). If so, identify the diagnosis or condition related to the target outcome(s) that have the most relevance to your agency.

_____

_____

- Do best practice recommendations exist for this diagnosis or condition?

_____

---

## AGENCY APPLICATION:

### Improving OASIS Outcomes through a Care Pathway *(continued)*

- Have you identified any additional standards of care through PI initiatives that will likely help to improve targeted outcome(s)? If so, list these:

  _____

  _____

  _____

  _____

- In addition to OASIS outcome indicators, develop agency supplemental outcome indicators that relate to patient/caretaker skills, knowledge, and compliance that are needed for self-management of the condition or diagnosis. List these:

  _____

  _____

  _____

  _____

---

2c

## INTEGRATING CARE PATHWAY OUTCOMES DATA INTO CLINICAL PRACTICE AND AGENCY OPERATIONS

Care pathway outcomes are integrated into everyday clinical practice and agency operations by first aggregating data retrospectively to the level of your primary patient population(s). Aggregating to the diagnosis helps to *drill down* the specifics associated with it. These aggregates help you pinpoint areas in need of improvement related to clinical interventions, efficiency and cost-effectiveness, staffing productivity and staffing mix, staff accountability, and staff competency. They can also form the basis of your marketing strategies, business and strategic planning, and should be an important factor in leadership decisions.

The following example demonstrates how aggregated, end-result outcomes from a total knee replacement pathway are integrated into practice and agency operation.

### Clinical Interventions and Quality of Care

Revisions in clinical interventions are made according to end-result outcomes achieved. Improvement in quality of care is determined over time by subsequent outcome measurements. For example, pathway outcomes show that 38% of this patient population had extreme joint stiffness and some complications the week following surgery. Investigation revealed that 82% of these same patients returned home Thursday afternoon or later, and were not evaluated by physical therapy until Monday. The joint replacement pathway was revised to include a therapy evaluation visit within 24 hours of the patient's return home.

This revision resulted in an improved quality of care for the patient as demonstrated by decreased stiffness and fewer unscheduled visits to the surgeon. Follow-up evaluation showed that only 8% had stiffness that required an unscheduled surgeon's office visit.

## Patient Satisfaction

Satisfaction improved as evidenced by the outcome of no complaints being made by patients and family. The satisfaction survey was revised to include the following element:

*I received timeliness of services according to my expectations.*

## Efficiency and Cost-Effectiveness

The revision in pathway standards of care improved the efficiency of therapy services provided. Patients needing a therapy evaluation and exercise received treatment in a timelier manner. The healthcare system cost-effectiveness was achieved by saving dollars previously spent for extra office visits and treatment, as well as for the small percentage of patients who were admitted to skilled care for intensive therapy.

## Staffing Productivity and Staff Mix

While revisions to the pathway were being considered, the therapy staffing mix and schedule were reviewed to determine if these issues affected this outcome. It was determined that two additional therapists were needed to provide adequate coverage for PT evaluations conducted on Fridays and treatment that begins on Saturdays or Sundays.

## Staff Accountability

Investigation of this outcome clearly demonstrated a problem in communication among therapists who were contracted individually by the agency. If all therapists' schedules were full on Friday, the patient was simply scheduled for Monday, believing that the patient would perform the exercises begun during hospitalization until the homecare therapist arrived. No policy existed regarding specific coverage in this instance. Subsequent to this investigation, a policy was written to address this issue. The therapy contract was amended to include Saturday and Sunday coverage.

## Staff Competency

Staff competency was determined not to be a contributing factor to this outcome.

## Marketing and Business

The agency communicated the improvement in patient outcomes to the orthopedic surgeons who use their services, two of whom previously called agency management to complain when patients returned to their offices unexpectedly with decreased mobility and function. These surgeons had decreased their admissions to the agency because of these occurrences.

Because the agency was able to demonstrate a considerable improvement in outcomes for these patients, it began to consider designing a special program for patients undergoing joint replacement. They enlisted the consultation of one of the orthopedic surgeons, who was particularly impressed with their improved outcomes.

Marketing strategies included the promotion of patients' preference of getting restorative treatment and aggressive therapy in their own home as opposed to additional days spent in a skilled-care facility. Providing therapy in the home also afforded the therapist the opportunity to assess the patient's home environment for potential safety issues and to teach the patient how to address these issues or maneuver around obstacles unique to patient's own environment.

---

### AGENCY APPLICATION:

### Integrating Outcomes into Care and Operations

Think of opportunities your agency has to integrate and use care pathway outcomes to improve the quality of services you provide.

_____

_____

_____

_____

_____

_____

2c

## REFERENCES

Centers for Medicare and Medicaid Services, U.S. Department of Health and Human Services. (Dec. 2002). Outcome-based quality improvement (OBQI) implementation manual. Baltimore, MD: author.

Cole, L., Houston, S., & Kite-Powell, D. (1995). *Developing and implementing outcomes-driven clinical pathways*. Nashville, TN: Business Network Inc.

Critical pathways—an acute care tool enters the home healthcare setting. (1994). *Hospital Home Health*, 11(1), 1–12.

Fuss, M. A. & Pasquale, M. D. (1998). Clinical management protocols: The bedside answer to clinical practice guidelines. *Journal of Trauma Nursing*, 5(1), 4–13. Retrieved May 16, 2003 from Infotrac database.

Gingerich, B. S. & Ondeck, D. A. (2001). *Clinical pathways for the multidisciplinary homecare team*. Gaithersburg, MD: Aspen.

Hazelip, J. (2002). Outcomes. *The Remington Report*, 10(6),10–13.

Hill, M. (1999). Outcomes measurement requires nursing to shift to outcome-based practice. *Nursing Administration Quarterly*, 24(1), 1–9. Retrieved January 8, 2003 from Infotrac database.

Humphrey, C. J. & Milone-Nuzzo. (1996). *Orientation to home care nursing*. Gaithersburg, MD: Aspen.

Joint Commission on Accreditation of Healthcare Organizations. (2004). *Comprehensive accreditation manual for home care: 2004–2005 camhc*. Oakbrook Terrace, IL: Joint Commission Resources.

Klenner, S. (2000). Mapping out a clinical pathway. *RN*, 63(6), 333.

Lagoe, R. J. (1998). Basic statistics for clinical pathway evaluation. *Nursing Economics*, 16(3), 125. Retrieved May 16, 2003 from Infotrac database.

Robert Luttman and Associates. (n.d.). Variance management systems. Retrieved June 1, 2003, from http://www.robertluttman.com/variance_short_take.html.

Matula, P. A. (1995). *Clinical paths: A practical approach to positive outcomes*. Nashville, TN: Business Network Inc.

Maturen, V. & Houser, N. (1994, May). Utilizing a managed care model to achieve cost and quality outcomes. Presented at the THERF Seminar. Tennessee Hospital Association, Nashville, TN.

*Merriam-Webster's Collegiate Dictionary (10th ed.)*. (2002). Springfield, MA: Merriam-Webster.

Polit, D. F., Beck, C. T., & Hungler, B. P. (2001). *Essentials of nursing research: Methods, appraisal, and utilization*. Philadelphia: Lippincott.

Sidorov, J., Shull, R., Tomcavage, J., Girolami, S., Lawton, N., & Harris, R. (2002). Does diabetes disease management save money and improve outcomes? *Diabetes Care*, 25(4), 684. Retrieved May 16, 2003 from Infotrac database.

Smith, A. P. (2001). Removing the fluff: The quality in quality improvement. *Nursing Economics*, 19(4), 183. Retrieved June 27, 2003 from Infotrac database.

Strassner, L. (1997). Critical pathways: The next generation of outcomes tracking. *Orthopaedic Nursing*, 16(2), S56. Retrieved May 16, 2003 from Infotrac database.

Waggoner, M. G. (1999). Clinical pathways: From the hospital to the home. *MedSurg Nursing*, 8(4), 265. Retrieved May 16, 2003 from Infotrac database.

# Building an Outcome-Based Approach to Home Care

# Disease Management (DM) and Outcome-Based Home Care

## CORE TERMS AND CONCEPTS

- Disease Management
- Disease Management Care Continuum
- Evidence-Based Guidelines
- Outcomes Management
- Patient Self-Care Management Education

## LEARNING OBJECTIVES

Upon completion of this topic, you will be able to:

1. Define Disease Management.
2. Describe contributions that are unique to home care in the disease management care continuum.
3. Identify diagnoses that are appropriate for disease management.
4. Outline the steps involved in developing and implementing a home care approach to disease management.

## AGENCY-SPECIFIC DATA/RESOURCES NEEDED

- Agency's primary patient population(s) and staff experience and expertise defined in Section A of this chapter

# INTRODUCTION

Interest and knowledge about disease management (DM) have grown dramatically (CMS, 2003) since the early 1990s, when a major paradigm shift began to evolve in health care. This was due in large part to fragmented care, financial pressures, the need for outcome-oriented quality improvement, and consumers demand for good care (Powell, 2001). Early efforts in DM occurred primarily in managed care settings, because plans and plan providers had clear incentives to manage care, and the patients were *enrolled* and *locked into* a health delivery system (CMS, 2003).

By the mid '90s, DM studies focused on cost-effectiveness and therapies in the practice setting (Epstein and Sherwood, 1996). Many of these studies demonstrated an improvement in patient outcomes and costs, and prompted healthcare providers of all types and third party payers to continue to study and refine DM implementation strategies.

Today, DM has emerged as a comprehensive, integrated approach to care and reimbursement based on the natural course of a disease. It focuses on wellness and prevention and ensures that patients are active participants in their own care (Waldo, 2000). New DM strategies are being implemented across the entire healthcare continuum to include multiple treatment modalities, such as nurse case management, telephonic and Internet communication and follow-up, clinical practice guidelines, and patient self-management (Greenberg, 2000; Sidorov, 2002).

The emphasis on providing DM across the healthcare continuum is a timely opportunity for homecare providers, who now have aggregated OASIS patient outcomes readily available for use. Patient and financial outcomes can be used to demonstrate home care's effectiveness in preventing complications, future hospitalizations and readmissions, and in describing factors affecting self-care management.

Recognizing the emergence of DM, two important entities have included it in their focus on healthcare. The Joint Commission on Accreditation of Healthcare Organizations (Joint Commission) now offers a Disease-Specific Care Certification program that recognizes high-quality DM programs ("DM certification," 2002; "Spotlight on new," 2002). The U.S. Department of Health and Human Services has funded DM demonstration projects beginning in 2003 ("Thompson pushes for," 2003). This section provides guidance for successful implementation of DM in the home care setting.

## WHAT IS DISEASE MANAGEMENT?

The Disease Management Association of America (DMAA) and The National Committee for Quality Assurance and other organizations, such as the National Pharmaceutical Council, have defined DM using certain common elements (CMS, 2003). These definitions view DM as *an approach to delivering health care to persons with chronic illnesses that aims to improve patient outcomes while containing health care costs* (CMS, 2003). Taft, Looker, and Cella (2000) describe the *ideal* DM condition as one that:

- is chronic and that lends itself to management,
- applies to a large population,
- generally incurs highly visible costs,
- has preventable use of healthcare resources,
- receives less attention than needed by healthcare providers,
- has the potential for having outcomes measured in a timely manner, and
- may have improved results through patient education and involvement in decision making.

# HOME CARE IN THE DM HEALTHCARE CONTINUUM

The homecare setting offers a unique opportunity for providers to play a significant role in DM (Knox and Mischke, 1999; Swavely, Peter, and Stephens, 1999). Two factors in particular have helped establish the important contribution that home care can make:

1. The prospective payment system (PPS) was initiated in 2000. PPS brought about several changes in home care that are required for a DM initiative. PPS-oriented software makes financial information available to *manage and lower* costs per episode specifically related to a patient's *primary diagnoses*. OASIS documentation results in *agency aggregated* outcomes that are benchmarked with a national reference sample, while OBQI encourages the use of *best practices* as a means of achieving better outcomes.
2. Providing care in the patient's residence affords advantages not found in other healthcare environments. Homecare providers can evaluate first hand the obstacles to *self-care management* faced by the patient and caretaker in their environment (Gorski and Johnson, 2003) and can more aptly assist the patient and family to remedy these as necessary. Noncompliance with treatment regimens can also be better understood and specific suggestions and assistance can be offered more appropriately to the patient's situation.

## DEVELOPING A SUCCESSFUL HOME CARE DM INITIATIVE

The DMAA (2003) states that DM primarily consists of:

- the identification of specific population(s),
- the use of evidenced-based practice guidelines,
- patient/family self-management education,
- collaboration among physicians, care providers, and support-service providers,
- outcome measurement, evaluation, and management,
- routine reporting and feedback loop.

The DMAA (2003) states that a full service DM program must have all six components as outlined above. Programs with fewer than six are considered *DM Support Services*. The following information briefly examines each of the primary elements in DM. Consider each element relative to its implementation in home care. Patient population(s) must be identified first. However, the remaining elements may be developed simultaneously or in any order.

### Identifying Specific Patient Populations

Disease management concentrates on chronic conditions that are typically difficult to manage, incur the greatest cost, and apply to a large segment of the population. The literature (CMS, 2002; Knox and Mischke, 1999; Sidorov, Shull, Tomcavage, Girolami, Lawton, and Harris, 2002; Taft, Looker, and Cella, 2000; Waldo, 2000) identifies several chronic conditions that are appropriate for DM:

- Congestive heart failure
- Coronary disease
- Stroke
- Hypertension
- Asthma
- COPD
- Diabetes
- Osteoporosis
- Arthritis
- Chronic wounds

*Guiding Questions*

- How many patients are admitted to the agency with these chronic diagnoses?
- What are the demographics of my patient population(s)? Average age?
- Who are the physicians and other practitioners who generally admit these patients to the agency?
- What are the co-morbidities, or secondary diagnoses, associated with the primary diagnoses?
- Are there preventative measures available to help manage the diagnoses? How effective are they?
- Which agency populations have the greatest potential for improvement in health-care outcomes?

---

## AGENCY APPLICATION:

### Selecting Diagnoses Appropriate for DM

Look at your agency's primary patient population(s) that you identified earlier in Section A of this chapter. Of these, identify the diagnoses that are appropriate for DM.

_____

_____

_____

Using those elements that describe the ideal disease management condition, does your agency have other diagnoses that fall into the realm of DM? If so, list these:

_____

_____

_____

Do any of the above diagnoses have high costs associated with treating them? Does it typically cost your agency more to treat the diagnosis than it receives in reimbursement?

From the previous basic information, prioritize the diagnoses that have the greatest potential for DM implementation in your agency:

1._____

2._____

3._____

## Using Evidence-Based Practice Guidelines

In Chapter 1, you learned how to locate evidence-based practice guidelines for the provision of care. These guidelines are a critical component in DM (AAFP, 2003; DMAA, 2003; "Disease management comes of age," 2002; Powell, 2001) because they generally yield better patient outcomes. Evidence-based practice typically includes screening and early detection, risk assessment, timeliness of diagnostics, prevention of complications and early reporting of signs and symptoms, patient compliance, patient self-management, and other clinical interventions, such as wound care, phlebotomy, administering injections, or infusion therapy. Many DM programs use care pathways.

Once you have selected the evidenced-based or best practice recommendations for a particular DM diagnosis, discuss these with your medical director/advisor or other physician customers who will be admitting patients with this diagnosis to your agency. The physician or other practitioner must have a sense of ownership and *commit* to the interventions you propose to use in order for DM to work (Wehrwein, 1997).

Now focus on your number one priority diagnosis for potential DM implementation. Review this *to do* list carefully and plan accordingly.

2D

1. *Learn all you can about the disease or condition and how it's treated* ("Select where you can have," 2002). Search for the latest sources of information.
2. *Gather and explore evidence-based interventions from valid health related sources* (Benefield, 2002; Rosswurm and Larrabee, 1999), such as clinical practice guidelines and recommendations of national organizations and associations.
3. *Evaluate the relevance of each intervention to the agency's population* (Benefield, 2002). For example, an exercise program probably has little relevance for the general population of severe end-stage COPD patients.
4. *Formulate your agency's best practice interventions for the DM diagnosis you have selected.*
5. *Re-evaluate staff competency based on best practice interventions that you plan to provide.* Determine skills competency assessment and training and education requirements that will be needed prior to implementation.
6. *Consider supply requirements and evaluate product lines as needed.* For example, in planning for a DM wound program, you discuss streamlining your product inventory with your medical advisor. You decide to stock no more than two product lines. Review supply costs and utilization. Make adjustments as needed.
7. *Evaluate the financial impact of interventions (Sidorov, 2003) by comparing costs versus average reimbursement per episode.* Figure the cost of interventions (cost per visit per discipline). Compare these with average reimbursement, realizing that care pathway interventions typically increase efficiency and lower overall costs. Include patient education tools, materials, and/or special monitoring devices in your costs. For example, you plan to include the use of photography and telephone follow-up on a weekly basis as a part of your intervention. Consider photography expenditures and also the time and labor required for your weekly phone calls. Conduct a follow-up financial evaluation at three and six months.
8. Determine how your documentation will change to incorporate best practice interventions necessary for the implementation of the DM care pathway.
9. Determine what type of support will be required of business office, clerical, and data entry staff to implement documentation requirements.

### Guiding Questions

- Have I exhausted the search for best practice guidelines?
- Are there other health professionals with expertise who can give guidance?
- Have agency referral sources been tapped for guidelines, if any, that they use?
- Do guidelines require competencies that will necessitate additional training?
- Does the agency have qualified individuals to conduct the training? Will outside resources be required?
- How will the pathway impact current methods of clinical documentation?

## AGENCY APPLICATION:

### Selecting Evidence-Based Practice Recommendations

Identify the DM diagnosis that your agency plans to explore first:

_____

Identify the individual(s) who will conduct the search for evidence-based practice recommendations:

_____

_____

List health-related sources that you plan to search for evidenced-based recommendations for this diagnosis (See Appendix A: Internet Resource Listing: Best
Practices):

_____

_____

_____

_____

_____

List all of the evidenced-based interventions that you find in your search and
the relevance of each to your patient population having this diagnosis:

Clinical Intervention                         Relevance

_____

_____

_____

_____

_____

_____

_____

Highlight the interventions that you propose to use.

# Patient/Family Self-Management Education

Self-care is *the practice of activities that individuals personally initiate and perform on their own behalf in maintaining life, health, and well-being* (Orem, 1971). Orem also states that action is deliberate when it is based on an *informed judgment* about the outcomes(s) resulting from a particular action. Learning how to self-manage through patient and family education can have a positive effect on patient outcomes, including compliance (Renders et al., 2001).

Patient self-management education is an integral part of the interventions that are implemented alongside best practice. For example, the Agency for Healthcare Research and Quality (AHRQ) clinical practice guideline for pressure ulcers includes patient risk assessment (DHHS, 2000). Not only do the clinicians perform a risk assessment on admission and periodically thereafter, but they teach the caretaker or family how to recognize when the patient is at increased risk.

Inadequate patient skills, knowledge, and motivation about self-care are important determinants of adverse health outcomes (Harris, 2000). According to research from the AHRQ (DHHS, 2002), people who self-manage their chronic diseases can prevent or delay disability, even in patients with heart disease, hypertension, or arthritis.

The Chronic Disease Self-Management Program, developed at the Stanford University Patient Education Research Center with AHRQ funding, teaches patients to control symptoms through a variety of self-management interventions. The program showed improvement in a variety of health-related conditions, including fewer visits to physicians and emergency departments ("Disease self-management can," 2002).

The DMAA (2003) recommends that DM self-management education include *primary prevention, behavior modification, and compliance/surveillance.*

## *Guiding Questions*

- Does our agency have the education tools to teach patients how to self-manage their chronic condition?
- Do we have standardized patient teaching materials for this diagnosis that include preventative measures, appropriate behavior modification strategies, and discussion of compliance issues?
- How do we include the caretaker or family in the instruction?
- Do staff need training in teaching patient self-management education?
- Does our agency have the resources and tools to conduct patient surveillance activities, such as follow-up phone calls during service or post discharge? Mail-out questionnaires? Internet contact? If not, how will we plan for this?
- Will our agency participate in a collaborative DM continuum that implements surveillance of the patient population via a provider, other than home care?

2D

## AGENCY APPLICATION:

### Selecting Interventions for Self-Management

*Use the DM diagnosis that your agency has decided to explore first.*
For each of the following elements, list the interventions that you plan to include in your DM approach:

*Primary prevention:* What prevention measures will we teach? What will our risk assessment be composed of? How will we instruct the patient/caretaker to recognize and report adverse signs and symptoms? Should they report problems first to the home health clinician or physician?

_____

_____

*Behavior modification:* List types of behavior modification techniques suitable for patients that are particularly useful in relation to the diagnosis we have chosen.

_____

_____

_____

*Compliance*: Does the health literature point out certain compliance issues particular to our diagnosis that the patient is likely to face? List these.

_____

_____

_____

*Surveillance*: How will we determine if the patient is being compliant with self-management? Will we measure compliance outcomes? Will we conduct telephone (Greenberg, 2000) or other follow-up contact to encourage compliance with treatment regimens?

List the method(s) that your agency will consider, as applicable.

_____

_____

_____

## Collaborating with Physicians, other Referral Sources, and Support Service Providers

Coordination between levels and sites of care and between different care providers has enhanced DM (AAFP, n.d.). In developing a CHF DM program for Evanston Northwestern Healthcare, Knox and Mischke (1999) reported that a multidisciplinary approach encompassing care across the continuum of inpatient, outpatient, and home care was advantageous to the patient and to the healthcare system.

By its nature, collaborative practice helps to keep the patient as the central focus of our efforts. For example, a hospital has implemented a DM program for inpatients admitted with a new diagnosis of asthma. However, the homecare agency that provides care to this same group of patients is not aware of the hospital's new program and practice guidelines for asthma and provides usual care to this patient group. The hospital evaluates its outcomes data over six months for emergent care utilization of asthma patients and finds it to be higher than expected. Based on the investigation of this outcome, it is determined that collaboration with the homecare provider and local outpatient pulmonary rehabilitation clinic is essential to improving this hospitalization outcome.

### Guiding Questions

- Do our physicians and other practitioners responsible for the plan of treatment agree to support our interventions? Some of the interventions?
- Do hospitals, outpatient clinics, skilled care facilities, etc. have DM or specialty programs that would benefit by having our agency be a part of the DM care continuum?
- Is our agency ready to ask for an appointment with the coordinator of the DM program(s) to determine if we can participate in this continuum of care? Are we prepared to explain what our agency has to offer, i.e., measurement of outcomes? Best practice interventions? Patient/caretaker self-management education include prevention strategies, behavior modification, and compliance?

---

### AGENCY APPLICATION:

#### Identifying Existing Local DM Continuums

Do any of your agency referral sources, such as hospitals, outpatient clinic(s), or MCOs, have DM programs? If so, list the referral source(s) and DM program(s):

_____

_____

_____

If not, is there potential to develop a DM approach through local collaborative efforts?

_____

## Outcome Measurement, Evaluation, and Management

A central theme of DM is outcomes management (Epstein and Sherwood, 1996). Outcomes give healthcare providers the information to manage a patient with a particular disease in terms of quality of care provided, cost-effectiveness, and quality of life. For example, one group of researchers studied the outcomes of patients with pneumonia and developed a way for clinicians to determine which patients with pneumonia could be treated safely at home (CMS, 2000). This option allowed for a reduction in Medicare costs and was preferred by many patients over hospitalization.

Once outcomes have been measured and aggregated, they are analyzed and trended to determine which outcomes have improved, worsened, or remained the same, as well as if the outcome measure is appropriate to the intervention. Depending upon these findings, revisions in care assessment and interventions are made. These revisions may call for a change in clinical documentation format, a re-evaluation of financial impact, intensified staff education efforts, elevated or revised staff competency, and/or a re-evaluation of overall program components.

There are times when an agency discovers that an outcome measure is not capturing the information it originally targeted and needs revision. In this case, do not hesitate to re-evaluate the outcome itself and revise it as needed. However, outcomes data should be collected over several months to a year before deciding that the outcome itself legitimately needs revision. When outcomes are properly written, measured accurately, and are appropriate to intervention(s), they may require only minor adjustments over the course of time.

An agency chooses how many and what type of outcome indicators to measure. When using OASIS-generated outcomes, an agency only has to select the outcomes that have relevance to the DM diagnosis or condition, as OASIS software calculates the measurement for you. You are encouraged to incorporate both OASIS outcomes and agency supplemental outcome measurements in your DM initiative.

Using both equips you with a well-rounded body of information to plan, implement, and review and revise your DM program. Agency supplemental outcome indicators give you the capability of measuring or tracking patient compliance and measuring knowledge acquired for essential patient self-management.

These indicators allow you to measure outcomes of particular interest for your referral sources. For example, the physicians who refer a large number of CHF patients to your agency use ace inhibitor therapy in the management of their patients, while others do not. These physicians want to know how well their patients adhere to this medication regimen. You write and measure an agency outcome indicator related specifically to this patient self-care management intervention.

Valid and reliable OASIS outcome measures indicate the improvement or decline in the patient's functional capability and clinical response to treatment, such as pain frequency, status of wounds, and dyspnea, all of which can severely impede patient progress. OASIS also captures adverse events that occur while patient is on service. OASIS outcomes allow for internal and external benchmarking, a function in DM that is necessary for evaluating your overall program in relation to others.

### Guiding Questions

- What are the outcomes that will be measured specific to your DM diagnosis?
- What are the OASIS outcomes that relate to the DM diagnoses you have chosen?
- Do the outcomes you are going to measure correlate with the best practice guidelines that you intend to implement?
- Do your referral sources measure outcomes for like diagnoses? If so, is there a way to collaborate with referral sources to share outcome findings to improve the continuum of care for the patient and family? Patient's quality of life? Market share? Cost-effectiveness?
- What are the outcomes that pertain to each discipline that will be providing care for patients with the DM diagnosis?

**AGENCY APPLICATION:**

**Selecting DM Outcome Indicators**

List the outcome indicators that the agency will measure related to your first listed DM diagnosis.

*Note: The number of blank lines provided does not indicate the number of outcomes you must measure.*

Agency written outcomes:

1. Patient/caretaker demonstrates _____

2. Patient/caretaker describes/verbalizes/identifies_____

3. Patient/caretaker is compliant with _____

4._____

5._____

6._____

7._____

8._____

9._____

10. _____

OASIS outcomes:

1._____

2._____

3._____

4._____

5._____

## Routine Reporting and Feedback Loop

Routine reporting and feedback can be accomplished through communication with patients, physicians, other practitioners involved in the patient's care, the patient's health plan, and ancillary providers (DMAA, 2003). An agency can start by identifying the individuals who will be part of the DM loop and discuss with them the types of information they need or prefer, its priority, and in what format. Consider the DM information that is used specifically to help achieve improved outcomes with less cost. The mechanism can be written, verbal, electronic, telephonic, and/or computerized.

- Discuss with the patient and caretaker the outcomes that will be measured and determine the goals that they want to achieve. Review interventions, including compliance.
- Report diagnostic results in a timely manner as appropriate to the findings. Patient progress should be communicated as frequently as needed to afford timely changes in treatment.
- Provide health plan coordinators with periodic progress updates and consider sharing outcomes achieved.
- Communicate patient needs appropriately to ancillary providers to help them deliver their products and services efficiently.
- Determine when outcome reports will be shared and what outcomes data are needed among providers in the loop.

*Guiding Questions*

- Who are the individuals in the agency's DM loop for the diagnosis you have chosen?
- What outcomes will our agency share with these individuals?
- What information will be routinely shared with the patient/caretaker by providers?
- Should we use periodic meetings or conferences to share overall successes, concerns, and issues related to the shared DM process?

---

### AGENCY APPLICATION:
### Identifying Your DM Feedback Loop

Identify the individuals in your DM feedback loop:

1. Patient and caretaker/family

2._____

3._____

4._____

5._____

6._____

7._____

8._____

9._____

10. _____

## AGENCY APPLICATION:

### Identifying Your DM Feedback Loop *(continued)*

Identify the patient information that you plan to provide to the patient and to other providers in your agency's DM loop.

Patient:

1._____

2._____

3._____

4._____

5._____

Providers:

1._____

2._____

3._____

4._____

5._____

6._____

7._____

8._____

9._____

10._____

2D

## REFERENCES

American Academy of Family Physicians. (2003). Policy and advocacy: Disease management. Retrieved April 16, 2003 from http://www.aafp.org/x6710.xml.

American Association of Family Practitioners. (n.d.). A position paper on disease management. Retrieved November 11, 2002 from Infotrac database.

Benefield, L. (2002). Evidence-based practice: Basic strategies for success. *Home Healthcare Nurse*, 20(12), 803–807.

Centers for Medicare and Medicaid Services, U.S. Department of Health and Human Services. (2003). Medicare program demonstration: Capitated disease management for beneficiaries with chronic illness [notice]. *Federal Register*, volume 68, number 40, Friday 28, 2003 p. 9673. Retrieved April 25, 2003 from http://www.cms.hhs.gov/healthplans/research/dmfinal.pdf.

Disease Management Association of America. (2003). Definition of disease management. Retrieved April 25, 2003 from http://www.dmaa.org/definition.html.

DM certification available from JCAHO: program assesses disease-specific care. (2002). *Case Management Advisor*, 13(5), 57. Retrieved April 16, 2003 from Infotrac database.

Disease management comes of age, not a moment too soon. (2002). *Medical Benefits*, 19(14), 5. Retrieved April 14, 2003 from Infotrac database.

Disease self-management can delay disability. (2002). Case management can delay disability. *Case Management Advisor*, 13(8), S1. Retrieved April 16, 2003 from Infotrac database.

Epstein, R. S. & Sherwood, L. M. (1996). From outcomes research to disease management: A guide for the perplexed. *Annals of Internal Medicine*, 124(9), 832–837. Retrieved April 16, 2003 from Infotrac database.

Gorski, L. A. & Johnson, K. (2003). Disease management program for heart failure. *Home Healthcare Nurse*, 21(11), 734–743.

Greenberg, M. E. (2000). Telephone nursing: Evidence of client and organizational benefits. *Nursing Economics*, 18(3), 117. Retrieved January 1, 2003 from Infotrac database.

Harris, M. I. (2000). Health care and health status and outcomes for patients with type 2 diabetes. *Diabetes Care*, 23(6), 754. Retrieved January 8, 2003 from Infotrac database.

Knox, D. & Mischke, L. (1999). Implementing a congestive heart failure disease management program to decrease length of stay and cost. *Journal of Cardiovascular Nursing*, 14(1), 55. Retrieved January 13, 2003 from Infotrac database.

Orem, D. (1971). *Nursing: Concepts of practice*. New York: McGraw Hill.

Powell, S. K. (2001). *Advanced case management: Outcomes and beyond*. Philadelphia: Lippincott.

Renders, C. M., Valk, G. D., Griffin, S. J., Wagner, E. H., Eijk Van, J. T., & Assendelft, W. J. J. (2001). Interventions to improve the management of diabetes in primary care, outpatient, and community settings. *Diabetes Care*, 24(10), 1821. Retrieved January 8, 2003 from Infotrac database.

Rosswurm, M. A. & Larrabee, J. H. (1999). A model for change to evidence-based practice. *Image: Journal of Nursing Scholarship*, 31(4), 317. Retrieved January 8, 2003 from Infotrac database.

Select where you can have impact on cost, utilization: Develop your DM program one step at a time. (2002). *Case Management Advisor*, 13(5), 51. Retrieved April 16, 2003 from Infotrac database.

Sidorov, J. (2002). Disease management is not only here to stay but it's bigger than you realize. *Physician Executive*, 28(6), 22. Retrieved April 16, 2003 from Infotrac database.

Sidorov, J. (2003). Building your own DM initiative. Feature lecture presented at the Disease Management Association of America 2003 Conference. Retrieved June 14, 2003 from http://www.dmaa.org/2003conference/sidorov.pdf.

Sidorov, J., Shull, R., Tomcavage, J., Girolami, S., Lawton, N., & Harris, R. (2002). Does diabetes disease management save money and improve outcomes? *Diabetes Care*, 25(4), 684. Retrieved April 16, 2003 from Infotrac database.

Spotlight on new disease-specific care certification program. (2002). *Patient Care Management*, 17(8), 6. Retrieved May 18, 2003 from Infotrac database.

Swavely, D. A., Peter, D. A., & Stephens, D. (1999). Improving smooth sailing between hospital and home. *MedSurg Nursing*, 8(5), 304. Retrieved April 16, 2003 from Infotrac database.

Taft, L. B., Looker, P., & Cella, D. (2000). Osteoporosis: A disease management opportunity. *Orthopaedic Nursing*, 19(2), 67. Retrieved January 8, 2003 from Infotrac database.

Thompson pushes for Medicare DM. (2003). *Medicine & Health*, 57(4), 5. Retrieved April 16, 2003 from Infotrac database.

U.S. Department of Health and Human Services. (2000). Outcomes research. [AHRQ Fact Sheet]. Retrieved April 24, 2003 from http://www.ahrq.gov/clinic/outfact.htm.

U.S. Department of Health and Human Services. (2002). Research in action: Preventing disability in the elderly with chronic disease (AHRQ, Issue No. 3). Retrieved April 25, 2003 from http://www.ahrq.gov/research/elderdis.pdf.

Waldo, B. (2000). Disease management gains acceptance—and finds its legs—with automation. *Nursing Economics*, 18(4), 208. Retrieved May 18, 2003 from Infotrac database.

Wehrwein, P. (1997). Disease management gains a degree of respectability. *Managed Care*. Retrieved June 14, 2003 from http://www.managedcaremag.com/carearchives/9708/9708.mainstream.html.

# CHAPTER 3

# Integrating Standards of Care and Outcomes into Staff Competency and Performance

# Competency Assessment: A Link to Outcomes Achieved

**CORE TERMS AND CONCEPTS**

- Clinical Competency
- Competency Indicator
- Competency Statement

## LEARNING OBJECTIVES

Upon completion of this topic, you will be able to:

1. Define clinical competency.
2. Incorporate best practice interventions into the competency assessment.
3. Link the competency assessment to clinical outcomes.
4. Develop or select appropriate methods of competency measurement.
5. Use competency aggregation to determine clinical competency needs and readiness.

## AGENCY-SPECIFIC DATA/RESOURCES NEEDED

Staff Experience and Expertise Survey from Chapter 2, Section A
Agency's OBQI Adverse Event report for the past 12 months
Agency's current competency assessment for RN/SN, HHA, PT/OT

# INTRODUCTION

In response to the changing healthcare environment, the way we assess clinical competence is changing. As our roles in relation to the provision of outcome-based home-care change, our traditional competency assessment will no longer suffice. The competency assessment must be linked to clinical outcomes, not just the ability to perform a particular task (Schroeder, 1997). Parsons and Capka (1997) and Schroeder (1997) point out that it is increasingly important to assess what the clinician *actually* does, not necessarily what one *is able to do*, as this can potentially affect the outcomes of the patient.

We now recognize that *knowing does not always equate with doing* (McGuire and Weisenbeck, 2001). It is not enough to know that providers are capable of safely carrying out a procedure; we must also demonstrate that when the procedure is carried out in the actual clinical setting, the patient outcomes reflect safety as well (Schroeder, 1997). When the clinician's competency improves, it is likely that positive patient outcomes most likely increase (Parsons and Capka, 1997; Rhetoric, 2001). Therefore, it only makes sense for the competency assessment to include essential elements that support the agency's desired clinical outcomes.

This section defines competency and explores the development of a competency assessment based on agency standards of care and desired outcomes. It concludes by describing how to use the aggregation of agency competency assessments to make decisions regarding the provision of outcome-based care delivery.

## WHAT IS CLINICAL COMPETENCY?

The majority of contemporary definitions of competency emphasize the outcome. This is significant because of the current healthcare outcome-oriented climate (Parsons and Capka, 1997). Competency is defined by Parsons and Capra as an outcome, as the *demonstrated ability to perform an identified cohort of skills in real situations*. They further clarify the definition to include the successful performance of key job functions, core skills, and behaviors specific to the responsibilities of the position and assigned duties.

Waddell (2001) describes competency as *an outcome of how proficiencies are used to reach performance goals*. The American Nurses Association (ANA, 1994) defines it as *the demonstration of knowledge and skills in meeting professional role expectations*. The Joint Commission on Accreditation of Healthcare Organizations (Joint Commission, 1997) defines competency as *a determination of an individual's capability to perform*, with capability being assessed, *demonstrated*, and improved.

## CLINICAL COMPETENCY AND ITS RELATIONSHIP TO PATIENT OUTCOMES

How should standards of care relate to the demonstrated competencies we choose to assess?

How should the competency assessment relate to patient outcomes we wish to achieve?

The competency assessment should focus on the clinician's ability to demonstrate the knowledge, skills, or behaviors necessary to implement the agency's best practices and standards of care. When designed with this in mind, the competency assessment becomes a management tool to:

- enhance staff accountability with patient outcomes achieved,
- educate staff to essential best practices and standards of care, and to
- provide planned opportunities for staff in need of skills remediation.

Patient populations served (Joint Commission, 2003) and best practices should be used by managers to prioritize essential content areas for the competency assessment. Note the following examples:

*Example 1*

The agency has a primary population of patients with malignant neoplasm. The latest OBQI outcome report indicates that this agency has a higher percentage of patients with intractable pain than the national average. There are two groups of oncologists in the area who have begun to admit patients to the agency. These oncologists use a specific pain protocol for patients in the home setting. Controlling pain is a major concern of the agency, as most of these patients will transition to palliative care, and the volume of this patient population is likely to remain steady or to increase due to the new physician referral sources.

In addition to the OASIS outcome: *Improvement in pain interfering with activity*, the agency has written and currently measures its own supplemental outcome for pain relief. It states: *Pain is managed or controlled to the patient/caretaker's level of satisfaction.* The agency designs one of its competency measures for medication administration specific to the physician's protocol for pain management. The competency includes proper use and implementation of the pain protocol.

*Example 2*

The agency has a large patient population with diabetes. One out of seven has difficulty seeing and has no one caretaker to assist with performing a finger stick glucose. Glucometer calibration and high and low controls are performed in a timely manner only 60 percent of the time. The staff use agency-provided glucometers.

Through performance improvement activities, the agency determined that one glucometer was easier to calibrate, thus enhancing staff compliance with timeliness of calibration, performing controls, and subsequent documentation; all standards of care that are critical to proper treatment, patient safety, and meeting accreditation standards. The competency assessment was amended to require the clinician to accurately calibrate and operate this agency glucometer with 100% accuracy, as well as to perform high and low controls. The assessment also requires the clinician to correctly document calibration and controls.

**3**A

*Example 3*

The agency's OASIS outcome percentages for *Emergent care for wound infection, deteriorating wound status*, and *Increase in number of pressure ulcers* are higher than the national average. This competency is related to the clinician's ability to demonstrate proper management of pressure ulcer prevention and treatment. Items in the competency assessment are developed based on the specific agency-desired outcomes for this patient population. To develop these items, managers address the following questions:

- What do the staff need to achieve the outcome of a decrease in pressure ulcers?
- Do staff accurately assess OASIS data set items related to pressure ulcers?
- Do staff know how to stage a pressure ulcer correctly, in order to recommend treatment accordingly?
- What are the best practices related to patients with pressure ulcers?
- What are the most important competencies related to these best practices that help achieve desired patient outcomes?

The agency has recently researched a clinical practice guideline for pressure ulcers. From the interventions included in the guideline, the agency outlines essential competencies for pressure ulcer care according to staff need. These include:

- *Accurate assessment of OASIS data set items, M0450, M0460, and M0464, according to definition.* Staff are required to state or recognize definitions with 100% accuracy.

- *Accurate calculation of an individual's risk assessment score using the Braden Scale.* Staff are given actual, current patient scenarios for which to apply the risk assessment scale. Staff must achieve 100% accuracy.
- *Proper identification of stage I, II, III, and IV pressure ulcers.* Staff are required to recognize the four stages of pressure ulcers from actual photographs with 100% accuracy.
- *Identification of wound cleansing and dressing appropriate to stage.* Staff are asked to select appropriate wound products according to stage with 100% accuracy.

---

## CONCEPT APPLICATION:
### Improving Outcomes through Clinical Competence

An agency wants to participate in a hospital-home care disease management (DM) continuum of care for congestive heart failure. However, the agency is concerned about its OASIS outcome: *Improvement in dyspnea*. It wants to improve this outcome before entering a DM relationship with its local medical center. After investigating this target outcome, the agency concludes that nursing and therapy staffs assess *M0490* somewhat differently and that nurses do not consistently discern rales or crackles from ronchi.

The agency designs education sessions for nursing that will use audio and videotapes, a practicum with a local nurse practitioner, and patient scenarios requiring accurate assessment of *M0490*. They also adopt the use of the hospital's dyspnea scale to assist the patient in describing his or her shortness of breath. Because dyspnea is often exacerbated during exertion when bathing, dressing, and exercising, the agency develops a learning module for home health aides and therapists that includes the use of the dyspnea scale and timely recognition of dyspnea that requires reporting.

The agency includes the following in the competency assessment of each discipline:

- Skilled Nurse: Recognition of rales, ronchi, and wheezing with 100% accuracy. The nurse practitioner assesses each individual, provides remediation as needed, and provides competency results to agency managers.
- Therapist (PT/OT) and Home Health Aide: Explains use of dyspnea scale with 100% accuracy. The therapist and HHA recognize when to report dyspnea in three actual patient scenarios with 100% accuracy.

---

## DEVELOPING A COMPETENCY ASSESSMENT THAT SUPPORTS DESIRED OUTCOMES

When developing a competency assessment based on best practice and patient outcomes, an agency should consider six important elements. These are:

1. Determining the **dimensions of care** that are appropriate to the agency's patient populations (del Bueno, 1997; Parsons and Capka, 1997).
2. Reviewing the agency's **best practice interventions relative to desired outcomes** (Waddell, 2001).
3. **Identifying essential competency indicators** relative to best practice interventions (Bradley and Huseman, 2003; Tipson and Turner, 2002; Waddell, 2001).

4. Developing or selecting **appropriate methods of measurement** of these competency indicators (Campbell and MacKay, 2001; Waddell, 2001).
5. Deciding **how often clinician competency is evaluated and by whom** (Campbell and MacKay, 2001; Neary, 2000).
6. Periodic review and evaluation of the **continued appropriateness of competency indicators** (Fitzpatrick, 2002).

## Dimensions of Care

Competency assessment is based on a framework that includes multiple dimensions, such as technical, human, and conceptual (Chase, 1994), interpersonal and critical thinking skills (delBueno, 1997), and job functions, core skills, and behaviors (Parsons and Capka, 1997). As described here, dimensions involve the realm of how competency is assessed. Will the agency verify competency primarily through the clinician's use of critical thinking skills, implementation of correct procedure, written tests, patient interaction, or a combination of all four? The agency may select the dimensions that meet the demands of the specific practice setting, meet the requirements for providing safe, effective, and efficient care to the agency's patient populations, and achieve agency desired outcomes.

While you should consider the scope of the dimensions of care that you think are important early on, you can also determine these as you formulate the competencies. As you work through this process, your approach may change from one competency to another.

For example, psychiatric patient care competencies generally include skills related to developing and maintaining a therapeutic interpersonal relationship. Additionally, a particular depression measurement tool helps the clinician plan more appropriate care to achieve improved outcomes in this patient group. One competency is chosen that verifies the clinician's ability to use this instrument properly. In this case, the dimensions of care include a combination of interpersonal behaviors and a core skill of correctly using the depression instrument.

**3A**

## Reviewing Agency Best Practice Standards Relative to Desired Outcomes

The critical link between standards of care and outcomes achieved transcends into competency assessment as well. Standards identify the essential content areas or competencies for staff orientation and periodic evaluation (Dozier, 1998). For example, an agency has recently implemented aspects of a clinical practice guideline for the *prevention* of pressure ulcers (CMS, 2000). The guideline contains interventions that are recommended as an adjunct to clinical judgment to improve patient outcomes. The following list includes the guideline's interventions that are further clarified in the agency's recently adopted standards of care.

*Note: Some of the agency's specific standards of care are located in parentheses just below the guideline's recommended interventions.*

- *Risk assessment*
  - Use of a valid risk assessment tool
    (Use of the Braden scale)
  - Periodic use of
    (Perform risk assessment on admission, at recertification, and resumption of care.)
- *Skin care and early treatment*
  - Skin inspection
    (The home health aide inspects all bony prominences for signs of redness or non-blanching during every visit in which personal hygiene is performed.)

- Skin cleansing
- Avoiding dry skin
- Massage
- Exposure to moisture
- Friction and shear injuries
  (Clinicians delegate the use of particular transfer and positioning techniques to prevent friction and shear injuries. The home health aide assignment reflects these interventions.)
- Nutrition
  (Patient and caretaker are taught that added protein and calories are necessary for regeneration. A standardized patient teaching booklet contains the foods that are recommended and the amounts needed. Every patient who is determined to be at risk for a pressure ulcer receives the agency teaching booklet and instruction.)
- Mobility/activity
- *Loading and support surface*
  - Repositioning
  - Positioning devices
  - Pressure relief for heels
  - Side lying positions
  - Lifting devices
  - Pressure-reducing devices for beds
    (Clinicians identify available pressure-reducing devices for beds and recommend them according to patient need.)
  - Pressure from sitting
  - Pressure-reducing devices for chairs
    (Clinicians identify available pressure-reducing devices for chairs and recommend them according to patient need.)
  - Postural alignment

---

### CONCEPT APPLICATION:
### Relating Standards of Care to Clinical Competence

1. Review the previous agency standards given in parentheses for pressure ulcer prevention.
2. Consider each standard as it relates to a competency that can be assessed or verified for appropriate discipline(s).

#### Guiding Questions

- What are the best practices for the patient population in question?
- Are the standards of care we wrote specific enough to assess competencies?
- Have clinicians had difficulty in implementing a standard? If so, is this due to a lack of knowledge, ability, or skill?
- Which standards are critical in achieving certain outcomes that have special significance to the agency?

---

## Identifying Essential Competency Indicators

Consider your agency's mission and goals, standards of care, desired outcomes, staff productivity and efficiency, costs, and customer feedback when selecting competency indicators (Fitzpatrick, 2002; McAdams and Montgomery, 2003). Select indicators upon which employees' actions will have a significant effect; doing so links your operational priorities to staff accountability. This link gives staff and management clear targets for decisions regarding performance improvement activities that contribute to the agency's overall mission and goals (Fitzpatrick, 2002).

Remember that it is neither feasible nor sensible to assess a competency for every standard of care that you implement or outcome that you wish to achieve. Prioritize and select competencies that reflect skills, knowledge, and behaviors that you deem *essential* to the implementation of these standards, and consider using performance improvement tools (Joint Commission, 1994) to help you accomplish this task.

For example, the agency performance improvement and staff development coordinators are given the task of selecting essential skills to include in the agency's competency assessment for *pressure ulcer prevention*. Realizing that best practice provides the basis for their clinical interventions, they review the guidelines relative to the agency's pressure ulcer population, the practice setting, and any skills that have been troublesome to staff. They determine which disciplines are involved.

Then they prioritize the competencies to be assessed through the use of a *priority matrix*, a performance improvement tool. They design the matrix to include best practices in a column to the left side of the tool. They choose the descriptors that are most important and list these horizontally across the top. Respondents are asked to correlate each intervention with each descriptor by placing a checkmark in every column that *describes* the implementation of the standard in the practice setting. The standards with the greatest number of checkmarks are considered those of highest priority. Agency managers and other leadership staff are asked to further refine this list, as necessary. The standards with highest priority should be used to develop staff competency indicators.

Examine the following results of the agency's priority matrix.

### Figure 3.1  Priority Matrix for Selecting Competency Indicators

| Descriptors: | High Risk | High Volume | Correlates with Critical Outcome | Lack of Knowledge | Other | Non-Essential |
|---|---|---|---|---|---|---|
| **Standards of Care** | | | | | | |
| *Risk Assessment* | | | | | | |
| Use of a valid risk assessment tool | ✔ | | ✔ | ✔ | | |
| Periodic Use of | | | | | ✔ | |
| *Skin Care/Early Tx* | | | | | | |
| Skin inspection | | | | | | |
| Skin cleansing | ✔ | | | | | |
| Avoiding dry skin | | | | | | |
| Massage | | | | | | |
| Exposure to moisture | ✔ | | | | | |
| Friction and shear injuries | ✔ | | ✔ | ✔ | | |
| Nutrition | | | ✔ | | | |
| Mobility/activity | ✔ | | ✔ | | | |
| *Loading and Support Surfaces* | | | | | | |
| Repositioning | ✔ | | ✔ | | | |
| Positioning devices | | | | ✔ | | |
| Pressure relief for heels | | | | | | |
| Side lying positions | | | | | | |
| Lifting devices | | | | ✔ | | |
| Pressure-reducing devices for beds | | | | | | |
| Pressure from sitting | | | | | | |
| Pressure-reducing devices for chairs | | | | ✔ | | |
| Postural alignment | | | | | | |

NOTES

3A

The following standards were chosen as priorities for competency assessment. The disciplines involved are noted, as well as the rationale for the decision.

- **Use of a valid pressure ulcer risk assessment tool—SN/PT**
  *Rationale:* The clinical practice guideline recommends use of a valid risk assessment tool. The agency implemented its tool six months ago. It is not always completed, and the directions within the tool are not always followed. Physical therapists admit "PT only" patients to the agency and need to accurately complete the tool as well. If risk is not identified properly or in a timely manner, this can contribute to an increase in pressure ulcers.
- **Friction and shear injuries—SN/PT/HHA**
  *Rationale:* Few SNs and PTs understood the concept of friction and shear injuries. As a result, the HHA assignment typically lacked instruction from clinicians regarding special techniques to prevent this type of injury. Home health aides needed to be able to position, transfer, and turn the patient properly to prevent friction and shear injuries in those identified at risk.

## Methods of Measuring Competency

A clinical competency can be written as a *statement* (Bradley and Huseman, 2003; Eichelberger and Hewlett, 1999), expressed as a measure (Waddell, 2001), or described as an *indicator* (Hader, Sorenson, Edelson, and Bliss-Holtz, 1999). The terms competency statement, competency measure, and competency indicator are used interchangeably to denote a criterion that is used to assess or verify competence.

*\*Note: The term competency indicator will be used throughout the remainder of the text.*

It may be necessary to have a subset of criteria for a particular competency indicator. These criteria are single, discrete, observable behaviors that are mandatory for the acceptable performance of the designated skill. These are called *critical elements* (Luttrell, Lenburg, Scherubel, Jacob, and Koch, 1999). A collective set of criteria to assess overall competence is often called a *competency instrument or tool.*

When deciding how to assess or measure competency, one of your most important decisions is between that of *selecting* a valid and reliable instrument that is already available or *developing* a valid and reliable instrument of your own. Consider the primary advantages and disadvantages of each.

### Selecting a Competency Instrument

Many competency instruments have validity and reliability already established, thus saving time and labor costs in development. However, the primary disadvantage is that you must take time to choose an instrument that is appropriate to your clinical setting. This may be a difficult task, as an instrument may not cover the competencies that align with your agency's particular desired outcomes and standards of care. Some portions of the instrument may apply to your patient population(s), and some may not. Cost can also be a factor.

### Developing a Competency Instrument

The advantage of developing your own instrument(s) is that you can develop any number of indicators with the level of specificity that you need to address those competencies you deem necessary. You can also develop any number of instruments and use a variety of methods, such as written tests, demonstration of specific skills, observation in a simulated or actual practice setting, or response to actual patient scenarios (LaDuke, 2000).

For example, your agency has a large number of pressure ulcer patients. Clinicians have difficulty using the agency's pressure ulcer risk assessment tool. You can develop a competency indicator to assess the skill of the clinician in the specific use of this tool.

NOTES

You can also write the competency indicator to elicit certain skills and knowledge that are problematic to the clinician (Willard, 2002). Then, you can use the competency instrument as a critical adjunct to performance improvement efforts and to enhance staff accountability with agency standards and expectations. When used in this way, the competency assessment becomes a part of the continuous circle of performance improvement.

Validity and reliability must also be established for competency indicators. The activities that establish the validity and reliability of outcome indicators are the same as the ones used for competency indicators.

## Writing Measurable Competency Indicators

Let's examine two recommendations from a clinical practice guideline that were prioritized from the performance improvement matrix and the disciplines involved.

Use of a valid pressure ulcer risk assessment tool—RN/PT/OT
Prevention of friction and shear injuries—SN/PT/HHA

*First*, prepare a draft of each competency indicator. Consider who, what, when, where, and how, as applicable. Focus on skills necessary to provide agency standards of care and those that help to achieve agency-desired outcomes. Prioritize these for inclusion in the competency assessment.

*Second*, re-examine the indicator or statement and determine if it is written as clearly as possible, so that no misunderstanding occurs on the part of the assessor or those being assessed. This may mean that you provide written definitions for each indicator, or other instructions as needed.

*Third*, re-examine each indicator and the accompanying instructions to determine if the skill, knowledge, or behavior that you intend to assess is actually being assessed. A thoughtful re-examination enhances your objectivity and clarity.

**3**A

# CONCEPT APPLICATION:
## Writing Measurable Competency Indicators

Using the previously discussed agency standards of care for prevention of pressure ulcers, study these measurable competency indicators designed to help achieve desired patient outcomes.

**Competency Indicator 1**

- **Standard/Discipline:** Use of a valid pressure ulcer risk assessment tool—SN/PT/OT.
  The problem with the risk assessment tool is lack of proper completion and follow-up. It is determined that the tool is somewhat difficult to use.

- **Indicators:**
  1. Skilled disciplines properly complete the agency pressure ulcer risk assessment tool.
  2. Appropriate follow-up is planned according to the agency standard.

- **Instructions:**
  1. A written, standard patient scenario is used. Clinician responses for the risk assessment are compared to acceptable, pre-printed responses for the scenario.
  2. The clinician must verbalize or write an appropriate plan for follow-up. This plan is likewise compared to acceptable, pre-printed responses for the scenario.

- **Scoring:**
  1. Clinician responses must align with those in the scenario to achieve *Satisfactory* competence.
  2. Scoring is the same as for 1.

**Competency Indicator 2**

- **Standard/Discipline:** Prevention of friction and shear injuries—SN/PT/HHA. Clinicians are unsure of techniques that help to prevent friction and shear injuries. Home health aides do not receive adequate instruction in the HHA assignment.

- **Indicators:**
  1. SN/PT (as appropriate) prepares adequate HHA instructions regarding positioning, transferring, and turning techniques that prevent shear and friction injuries.
  2. HHA demonstrates proper positioning, transferring, and turning techniques to be used for patients at risk, as directed by the HHA assignment.

- **Instructions:**
  The agency develops five standard techniques of positioning, transferring, and turning to help prevent friction and shear. These five techniques are the basis for the determination of competency.

- **Scoring:**
  1. The SN/PT (as appropriate)/HHA describes each of these five methods and gives appropriate instruction to receive a score of *Satisfactory*.
  2. The HHA must demonstrate each of these five methods to receive a score of *Satisfactory*.

## CONCEPT APPLICATION:
### Identifying Measurable Competency Indicators

Agency managers have prepared a list of competency indicators to support agency standards of care and achieve agency-related outcomes. However, some of these are not written objectively to attain this end. Identify which competency indicators *are not constructed objectively* by writing *No* in the corresponding blank.

_____ 1. Initiates vascular infusion according to agency protocol.

_____ 2. Demonstrates agency-approved hand washing technique using soap and water; waterless cleanser.

_____ 3. Administers medication appropriately.

_____ 4. Achieves a score of *Satisfactory* on the agency's OASIS Definitions Test.

_____ 5. Dons all appropriate apparel for *Contact* precautions.

_____ 6. Verbalizes agency's nutrition standard for patients with diabetes with 100% accuracy.

_____ 7. Implements agency skin care protocol.

_____ 8. Scores *Satisfactory* on agency's ICD-9 coding exam.

_____ 9. Properly auscultates lung sounds.

_____ 10. Plans for and teaches flexibility and stretching exercises for all patients 65 and older who receive physical and/or occupational therapy.

*Answers: "No" should be written for 3, 7, 9, & 10.*
*Rationale: These indicators do not have enough information within or do not have information that can be obtained elsewhere that allows for measurable action.*

**3**A

## AGENCY APPLICATION:
## Writing Measurable Competency Indicators

Write competency indicators appropriate for the following scenario:

Agency clinicians do not routinely assess for pressure reduction devices for beds or request orders for procurement. The agency has an OASIS outcome of *Increase in pressure ulcers* that is higher than the national average. Because new devices are frequently introduced to the market, agency managers want clinicians to be keenly aware of the type and availability, how to assess for patient need, and how to procure the device in a timely manner.

*Element within the AHRQ clinical practice guideline:*
  Pressure-reducing devices for beds

*Agency's standards of care:*

Clinician:

  • Assesses need for device according to risk assessment or presence of ulcer.
  • Places order for procurement within 48 hours of admission.

Using the agency's critical elements for implementation of the standards, write the following:

  • Competency indicator(s)
  • Applicable discipline(s)
  • Instructions to Users, as needed
  • Method(s) of scoring

**Competency Indicator(s)/Applicable Discipline(s):**

_____

_____

_____

**Instructions to Users:**

_____

_____

_____

**Method(s) of Scoring:**

_____

_____

_____

## AGENCY APPLICATION:
### Evaluation of Agency's Current Competency Assessment Tools

Review the indicators in your agency's current competency assessment for each discipline.

Place a checkmark by those indicators that you consider a priority, given your primary patient populations, practice setting, and the patient outcomes your agency desires to achieve.

Review how these are written, using the following guiding questions.

*Guiding Questions*

- Are definitions or instructions provided for the use of the assessment tool?
- For the use of each indicator, as needed?
- If not, are the competency indicators written so that the staff member being assessed and the individual conducting the assessment have no misunderstanding of how the indicators are measured?
- Do indicators assess the ability of the staff to demonstrate competence related to specific skills, behaviors, or knowledge required to implement standards of care and to achieve desired outcomes?
- If not, which indicators need review, revision, deleting, or replacing?

3A

## Determining the Frequency of Competency Assessment

Regulatory and accrediting bodies and some state boards for health professionals give requirements and guidance to homecare agencies regarding the minimum acceptable frequency of competency assessments and verification (CMS, 2000; Joint Commission, 2002). Accrediting and regulatory bodies require initial competency requirements, as well as acceptable standards for frequency of re-assessment. Some state boards require completion of a specific number of continuing education hours during a specified timeframe, while others accept license renewal as verification of continued competency.

Within these various requirements, an agency can determine how often competency is conducted for skills, knowledge, and behaviors that affect implementation of agency standards and outcomes achieved. The potential impact that staff competency has on patient outcomes (Dozier, 1998; Luttrell et al., 1999) and the use of competency in appraising employee performance make an *annual* assessment of competency a logical choice when determining its minimum frequency.

Reviewing patient outcome reports from quarter-to-quarter or month-to-month provides valuable insight into the skills and knowledge necessary to achieve improved patient outcomes. Conducting competency on at least an annual basis integrates well with a timely response that is recommended by the Centers for Medicare and Medicaid Services for OBQI performance improvement efforts (CMS, 2002).

**AGENCY APPLICATION:**

**Frequency of Competency Assessments**

What is your agency's current frequency for the competency assessment of each discipline?

Frequency

SN _____

PT _____

OT _____

HHA _____

MSS _____

Dietitian _____

*Guiding Questions*

- Is the frequency appropriate for enhancing skills, knowledge, and behaviors needed by staff to improve patient outcomes?
- Is the frequency appropriate given your staff turnover?

## Selecting Individuals to Perform Competency Assessment

Practitioners who know your agency's process for conducting competency should oversee your competency assessment program (Neary, 2000). These individuals are responsible for ensuring that competency indicators are adequately written to elicit measurable responses from staff. They should also be involved in assessing competence or coordinating and directing the efforts of others to assess or verify staff competence.

Any individual possessing the knowledge and skills to conduct the assessment may assess staff competence (Joint Commission, 2002), in accordance with law and regulation. This person may be a staff member with specific expertise, a supervisor, and/or someone from outside the organization; what is important is that the individual has the expertise to evaluate the skills being assessed (Joint Commission, 2002).

## AGENCY APPLICATION:
### Conducting the Competency Assessment

Who in your agency conducts the competency assessment for each discipline?

_____

_____

_____

Are these individuals the most appropriate ones to assess the competency of others? _____

If you need additional individuals to assist in evaluating competency, review your agency's *Staff Experience and Expertise Survey* from Chapter 2, Section A. From this survey, note the senior clinicians that have the expertise to evaluate the skills of others. Consider enlisting these individuals to assist with competency verification. Consider those outside the agency who are qualified.

List these names below.

1._____

2._____

3._____

**3**A

## Review and Evaluation of Continued Appropriateness of Competency Indicators

Because the competency assessment includes indicators that help support your agency's mission and goals, standards of care, and desired outcomes, it changes as your needs evolve and change. This does not imply that the assessment is in a constant state of revision. However, competency indicators do require periodic review and evaluation to determine continued appropriateness according to outcomes achieved. The agency determines how often revision occurs.

If you find that a competency measure does not have a significant impact on quality outcomes, stop measuring it (Fitzpatrick, 2002). Likewise, if the measure itself is not producing the appropriate competency to improve clinical outcomes, revise it.

For example, an agency currently verifies clinician competency of staging pressure ulcers through a written test based on the definitions of each stage found in the OASIS implementation manual (CMS, 2002). However, the investigation of the target outcomes *Increase in pressure ulcers* and *Emergent care for wound infection, deteriorating wound status*, reveals that staff are experiencing continued difficulty with staging a pressure ulcer. This difficulty seems to be affecting this outcome. The agency does not have access to a wound specialty nurse. The company that provides the majority of the agency's wound products has provided in-service education for the staff on two occasions during the past six months. New staff have also been hired during this time.

When thinking about this from an outcomes-perspective, agency managers consider the following:

- The problem is not limited to new staff or to any clinician(s) in particular.
- The current method of competency assessment is not affecting this outcome positively.
- Education sessions alone have not yielded the skills necessary to properly stage a pressure ulcer.
- The agency has no ready access to a wound specialty nurse.
- The agency outcomes *Increase in pressure ulcers* and *Emergent care for wound infections, deteriorating wound status* have not improved over the past six months, since education began.

The agency realizes that revising its competency assessment tool will help address this problem by assessing the actual skill required to stage a pressure ulcer. They decide to verify this competency by having the clinician identify the four different stages as shown in actual wound photos. Agency managers believe this method to be a more accurate way of assessing this competency and potentially improving the OASIS outcome *Emergent care for wound infections, deteriorating wound status.*

The agency revises its competency assessment. Assessing the clinician's knowledge of the definitions is replaced with assessing the ability to identify stages I, II, III, and IV pressure ulcers from actual wound photos. The agency uses its required annual program evaluation (CMS, 2000) as the vehicle through which a periodic evaluation of the agency's competency assessment indicators and tool(s) is summarized and related activities are reported.

---

### AGENCY APPLICATION:
#### Appropriateness of Agency Competency Indicators

1. Refer to your agency's current competency assessment for each discipline.

2. Evaluate each assessment's indicators relative to its appropriateness to your primary patient population(s), practice setting, and overall agency goals.

3. Place a checkmark beside those indicators that need review, revision, or deletion.

4. What revisions or deletions are needed, if any?

_____

_____

_____

*Guiding Questions*

- Do the agency's competency assessments contain indicators that may improve agency outcomes?
- Are the competency indicators or critical elements objective enough to elicit the skills, knowledge, and/or behaviors needed to affect implementation of standards of care and desired patient outcomes?
- Who is most qualified to assess these competency indicators?
- *When* and *how* are staff made aware of the change in competence requirements?
- Who will provide the education?

## REMEDIATION OF UNMET COMPETENCY

Accrediting bodies for home care require that organizations take action to improve an individual's competence (Joint Commission, 2002). This can be prompted by individual assessment findings or from aggregated data from performance improvement activities. To improve competence, a scoring mechanism must designate when improvement through remediation is required. Each competency indicator is designated as Met or Unmet, Satisfactory or Unsatisfactory, Acceptable or Unacceptable. Other notations may be used to denote the measurement or score that the individual attains. Remediation may be conducted in a number of ways, as long as they support implementation of standards of care and achieve desired patient outcomes.

1. Provide education at the time of assessment, allowing the individual another opportunity to assimilate the concepts and re-apply them correctly. This means that the person who is assessing has the knowledge and expertise to educate on the subject, not only to determine a score.
2. Knowledge deficits that are not easily managed following assessment may require remedial work at another time. This may include self-instruction materials, formal classes, brief in-service opportunities, or a clinical practicum on or off-site. These opportunities should be planned ahead so that staff know what the remediation entails and the time that is required. Upon completion of the remedial work, competency is re-assessed.
3. There are occasions when unmet competencies are best managed by the individual's first line supervisor or by the director. In this case, the unmet competency may involve a compliance issue and not lack of knowledge (Bradley and Huseman, 2003).

## AGGREGATION AND ANALYSIS OF COMPETENCY MEASUREMENTS

**3A**

Aggregating and analyzing staff competency is a valuable tool in outcome-based quality improvement. Aggregation of competency measurements or scores follows the same method as outcomes aggregation. All scores for different disciplines are aggregated for various sets or subsets of skills, knowledge, and/or behaviors. Percentages are calculated.

Calculating competency percentages allows managers and directors to pinpoint any number of specific areas that need attention. For example, the clinical practice guideline for *Pressure Ulcer Prevention and Treatment* (DHHS, 2000) entails a significant number of skills. There may be certain areas in which staff have deficits and others where staff have particular strengths. Aggregating competency scores allows managers to determine how extensive and in what areas a deficit exists.

Aggregated percentages give managers information on which to base decisions regarding amount of training and education required, costs, risk management, quality of care issues, and to determine where competency deficits exist. Are only two or three staff members having difficulty and need remediation, or are several staff members struggling with implementing certain standards due to a specific skill or knowledge deficit? If several staff members are struggling with a particular competency, the competency needs to be reviewed for applicability. If the competency indicator is appropriate and applicable, the agency should provide needed education opportunities to remedy the deficit. If education does not resolve the need, staff accountability must be addressed.

## CONCEPT APPLICATION:
### Aggregating Competency Results

Let's refer to a previous example in which the agency prepares to enter an alliance with a local medical center to provide a DM continuum of care for CHF patients. Agency managers want to improve the competence of staff prior to entering the alliance. Over three months, agency managers provide intensive education and competency assessment to prepare staff. Upon completion, the agency director uses an *aggregation of competency measurements* to help determine readiness of staff. The overall percentage of competence is shown for each indicator. Remediation percentages indicating the percentage of individuals needing remediation are given to achieve the overall competency percentage.

The results are as follows:

| Discipline | SN | PT | OT | HHA |
|---|---|---|---|---|
| **Indicators** | | | | |
| Recognition of Reportable Dyspnea | — | 100% | 100% | 100% |
| *Remediation %* | | *3%* | *5%* | *3%* |
| Use of Dyspnea Scale | 100% | 100% | 100% | 100% |
| *Remediation %* | *0%* | *0%* | *0%* | *4%* |
| Recognition of Rales, | 97% | — | — | — |
| Rhonchi, | 94% | — | — | — |
| Wheezes | 100% | 100% | 100% | 100% |
| *Remediation %* | *5%* | — | — | — |

This aggregation of competency helps the agency director know the level of staff clinical preparedness related to these priorities at this point in time.

However, competency aggregation can be calculated at any time for all competency indicators for all disciplines; it can be limited to essential indicators for the preparation of a new service, as shown in the above example.

## AGENCY APPLICATION:
### Aggregation of Agency Clinical Competence

1. Review a sample of your agency's competency assessments for each discipline.

2. Determine if items or indicators are appropriate for measurement and scoring.

*Guiding Questions*

- Are measurements capable of being aggregated as a percentage for each discipline?
- Is the aggregated percentage evaluated with respect to agency goals and expectations of staff?
- Is the competency assessment aggregation included in the annual agency evaluation?

## REFERENCES

American Nurses Association. (1994). *Standards for nursing professional development: Continuing education and staff development.* Washington, DC: American Nurses Publishing.

Bradley, D. & Huseman, S. (2003). Validating competency at the bedside. *Journal for Nurses in Staff Development,* 19(4), 165–173.

Campbell, B. & MacKay, G. (2001). Continuing competence: An Ontario nursing program that regularly supports nurses and employers. *Nursing Administration Quarterly,* 25(2), 22. Retrieved September 4, 2003 from Infotrac database.

Centers for Medicare and Medicaid Services, U.S. Department of Health & Human Services. (2000). Conditions of participation: Interpretive guidelines—home health agencies [Appendix B]. Retrieved from http://www.cms.hhs.gov/oasis/intguide.pdf.

Centers for Medicare and Medicaid Services, U.S. Department of Health & Human Services. (2002). Outcome-base quality improvement (OBQI) implementation manual. Baltimore, MD: author.

Centers for Medicare and Medicaid Services, U.S. Department of Health & Human Services: Health Care Financing Administration. (2002). Outcome and assessment information set: Implementation manual. Washington, DC: author.

Chase, L. (1994). Nurse manager competencies. *Journal of Nursing Administration,* 24 (1994, April), 56–64.

del Bueno, D. (1997). Assuring continued competence: State of the science. *Online Journal of Issues in Nursing.* Retrieved from http://www.nursingworld.org/ojin/tpc3/tpc3_3.htm.

Dozier, A. M. (1998). Professional standards: Linking care, competence, and quality. *Journal of Nursing Care Quality,* (1998, April), 22.

Eichelberger, L. W. & Hewlett, P. O. (1999). Competency model 101. *Nursing and Health Care Perspectives,* 20(4), 204. Retrieved September 4, 2003 from Galenet database.

Fitzpatrick, M. A. (2002). Let's bring balance to health care. *Nursing Management,* 33(3), 35.

Hader, R., Sorenson, E. R., Edelson, W., & Bliss-Holtz, J. (1999). Developing a registered nurse performance appraisal tool. *Journal of Nursing Administration,* 29(9), 26–32.

Joint Commission on Accreditation of Healthcare Organizations. (1994). *Framework for improving performance: From principles to practice.* Oakbrook Terrace, IL: author.

Joint Commission on Accreditation of Healthcare Organizations. (1997). *Comprehensive accreditation manual for hospitals.* Oakbrook Terrace, IL: author.

Joint Commission on Accreditation of Healthcare Organizations. (2002). *Comprehensive accreditation manual for home*

*care.* Oakbrook Terrace, IL: Joint Commission Resources.

Joint Commission on Accreditation of Healthcare Organizations. (2003). *Comprehensive accreditation manual for home care: 2004–2005 camhc.* Oakbrook Terrace, IL: Joint Commission Resources.

LaDuke, S. (2000). Competency assessments. A case for the nursing interventions classification and the observation of daily work. *Journal of Nursing Administration,* 30(7–8), 339–340.

Luttrell, M. F., Lenburg, C. B., Scherubel, J. C, Jacob, S. R., & Koch, R.W. (1999). Competency outcomes for learning and performance improvement. *Nursing and Health Care Perspectives,* 20(3), 134. Retrieved September 4, 2003 from Infotrac database.

McAdams, C. C. & Montgomery, K. A. (2003). Narrowing the possibilities: Using quality improvement tools to decrease competence overload. *Journal for Nurses in Staff Development,* 19(1), 40–46.

McGuire, C. A. & Weisenbeck, S. M. (2001). Revolution or evolution: Competency validation in Kentucky. *Nursing Administration Quarterly,* 25(2), 31. Retrieved September 4, 2003 from Infotrac database.

Neary, M. (2000). *Teaching, assessing and evaluation for clinical competence: A practical guide for practitioners and teachers.* Great Britain: Stanley Thornes Ltd.

Parsons, E.C. & Capka, M.B. (1997). Building a successful risk-based competency assessment model. *AORN Journal,* 66(6), 1065. Retrieved September 4, 2003 from Infotrac database.

Rhetoric, E. S. (2001). Patients in stroke unit have better outcomes, but receive less personal nursing care. *Evidence-Based Nursing,* 4(4), 128. Retrieved September 4, 2003 from Infotrac database.

Schroeder, P. (1997). Are you linking competence to outcomes? *Journal of Nursing Care Quality,* 12(2), 1. Retrieved September 4, 2003 from Infotrac database.

Tipson, M. & Turner. E. (2002). Career and competency framework for diabetes nursing. *Journal of Diabetes Nursing,* 6(6), 179. Retrieved September 4, 2003 from Galenet database.

U.S. Department of Health and Human Services. (2000). Clinical practice guideline: Pressure ulcers in adults. Agency for Healthcare Research and Quality. Retrieved from http://hstat.nlm.nih.gov/hq/Hquest/db/local.ahcpr.quickputq/screen.

Waddell, D. L. (2001). Management issues in promoting continued competence. *The Journal of Continuing Education in Nursing,* 32(3), 102-106.

Willard, M. J. (2002). Seeking a clinical competency tool. *Nursing Management,* 33(7), 6.

**3**A

# CHAPTER 3B

# Integrating Standards of Care and Outcomes into Staff Competency and Performance

## Section B

## Performance Appraisal: Accountability for Implementing Outcome-Based Care

> **CORE TERMS AND CONCEPTS**
>
> - Performance appraisal
> - Performance appraisal indicators
> - Outcome-based performance appraisal

### LEARNING OBJECTIVES

Upon completion of this topic, you will able to:

1. Describe the purpose of the performance appraisal in outcome-based patient care.
2. Describe the relationship between the outcome-based competency assessment and performance appraisal.
3. Develop performance appraisal indicators that reflect the agency's best practice standards of care and overall performance improvement goals.

### AGENCY-SPECIFIC DATA/RESOURCES NEEDED

Agency's current performance appraisal for each discipline

# INTRODUCTION

Just as competency indicators are changing to support an outcome-based approach to patient care, so is the performance appraisal. Past appraisal schemes tended to concentrate mainly on personal traits and behaviors that the individual displayed, such as loyalty, initiative (Beaumont, 1993), cooperation, and helpful attitude. More recently, the emphasis has turned to *job results*, or *what an individual achieves* (Beaumont, 1993).

The methodology of measurement is likewise shifting from general categories to specific objectives and criteria (Wiles and Bishop, 2001). When developed and written on this premise, the performance appraisal is a substantive tool for holding staff accountable for the implementation of agency standards of care, for lending foundational support to the agency's overall desired outcomes, for achieving performance improvement goals, and for providing salary increases for a job well done.

This section discusses the purpose of the performance appraisal, the relationship between the competency assessment and the performance appraisal, and how to develop performance appraisal indicators that support outcome-based care provision.

## PURPOSE OF THE PERFORMANCE APPRAISAL IN OUTCOME-BASED PATIENT CARE

There are three primary goals of the performance appraisal. They are:

- to provide an equitable measurement of an employee's contribution to the work force,
- to obtain a high level of quality and quantity of work produced, and
- to produce accurate appraisal documentation to protect both the employee and the employer (Capko, 2003).

In outcome-based patient care delivery, these goals change from generalities to specific results. These include overall agency results as well as individual results attained.

For example, the employee's *contribution to the work force* includes recognition of his or her contribution in achieving overall patient outcomes and enhancing processes and/or care delivery through performance improvement. A *high level of quality and quantity of work produced* involves the appropriateness and frequency for which agency standards of care are implemented. It also incorporates accuracy of assessment data that affect patient outcomes and agency financials. *Accurate appraisal documentation* includes specifics in measurable terms and the level at which the individual is held accountable. For example, RNs, LPNs, and HHAs have different levels of responsibility in preventing skin breakdown.

## THE RELATIONSHIP BETWEEN THE COMPETENCY ASSESSMENT AND THE PERFORMANCE APPRAISAL

The performance appraisal differs from the competency assessment in that competency evaluates whether an individual has the *knowledge, education, skills, and proficiency to perform assigned responsibilities*, whereas the performance appraisal evaluates *how well* an individual performs these assigned responsibilities (Herringer, 2002). When both competence and performance appraisal indicators are specifically designed to compliment each other, the result is a set of useful tools that help establish the expectations and accountability in outcome-based patient care.

The appraisal is an excellent vehicle for incorporating the results of an individual's competence, for noting progress or lack of progress with how well assigned tasks are implemented, and for giving the employee an opportunity to discuss his or her needs to improve identified deficits.

For example, the performance appraisal is typically administered at the end of orientation (6–12 weeks), the end of a probationary or conditional period (3–6 months), and annually thereafter (McAdams and Montgomery, 2003). Each time the appraisal is given, the employee's first-line supervisor takes the opportunity to discuss the level of competence that has been acquired up this point to implement agency standard of care and to achieve agency-desired outcomes. This not only allows necessary feedback between the manager and the employee, but also reinforces the agency's priority outcomes, the agency's overall goals related to outcome-based care provision, and more importantly, the role of the employee in helping to achieve them.

Essential competencies can be incorporated into the performance appraisal as direct individual measures or as a global measure for the individual's overall competence. For example, an agency has an important focus on pain management, as its primary patient population over the past two years involves orthopedics. The competency section of the performance appraisal addresses an individual aspect of pain management by indicating if the clinician manages pain according to the agency's pain protocol.

Another way of incorporating competence into the appraisal is by including a global measure that compares the individual's current level of competence to that of the last appraisal. A combination of both approaches can also be used. Many performance appraisals include a category related to Job Knowledge. This is an appropriate place to credit an individual's performance relative to competence.

## DEVELOPING OUTCOME-BASED PERFORMANCE APPRAISAL INDICATORS

An outcome-based performance appraisal not only evaluates an individual's accountability for implementing patient care standards and achieving clinical outcomes, but it also evaluates other attributes as well.

For example, the performance appraisal indicator *No pattern of tardiness or pattern of absence from work* is evaluated based on the employee's attendance record. The outcome of the employee's attendance, as measured by this indicator, denotes whether a pattern is evident or not and identifies if the employee is punctual. This employee performance *outcome* is measured without specific reference to the agency's patient outcomes.

Regarding outcome-based patient care, the performance appraisal need not contain a plethora of items that reflect all standards that are implemented or all outcomes that are measured; nor should it address all top primary diagnoses or patient populations. This is neither practical nor warranted. Select those that have the greatest impact on the quality of care that your staff provides and on agency performance improvement goals. Include indicators that have the greatest potential impact on outcomes that the agency deems a priority.

Consider the agency's practice setting, primary patient populations, and overall agency goals, and prioritize your standards of care and desired outcomes accordingly. These should be reflected in the appraisal as appropriate. Selecting or developing performance appraisal indicators follows the same process as that for competency indicators.

Indicators should reflect what, when, where, and how for each item and be written objectively for accurate measurement. Objective indicators are not always easy to develop. Be sure that the indicator is in fact, measurable. A good rule of thumb to test an indicator for objectivity is to examine whether it is written so the assessor can determine the score from documented records and reports, anecdotal notes, documented observation, and/or medical records.

The design of the outcome-based performance appraisal should *easily* accommodate the addition and elimination of items pertinent to changing priorities in care provision. Evaluate performance appraisals based on agency priorities and outcome-based goals at least every two years to determine the need for revision.

## CONCEPT APPLICATION:
### Basing Performance Indicators on Standards of Care

An agency has implemented a standard of care for patients with a pressure ulcer. The following indicators are excerpts from a performance appraisal for each associated discipline. This appraisal includes a section related to competence, entitled Job Knowledge.

*Note: Several indicators are provided as examples. This number does not imply that a proportionate number of indicators are required or recommended.*

**Registered Nurse**

*Quality*
- Consistently describes wound status according to agency-required indices. (Agency-specific)
- Recognizes wound deterioration and reports patient status promptly on the same day.
- Conducts planned, timely follow-up to risk assessment according to agency standard.
- Notifies physician when patient's wound does not respond to treatment. (Agency timeframe)
- Includes appropriate techniques for preventing friction and shear within the HHA assignment for all patients identified at risk for pressure ulcers.

*Quantity*
- Consistently submits completed OASIS assessments within _____. (Agency timeframe)
- Completes patient outcome measurements according to agency timeframes. (Agency-specific)

*Job Knowledge*
- Stages pressure ulcers with 100% accuracy.
- Scores Satisfactory on OASIS item instructions test.
- Measures a wound by length by width by depth 100% of the time.

**Registered Physical Therapist**

*Quality*
- Performs wound debridement without an adverse patient response. (State practice act permitting)

*Quantity*
- Submits completed OASIS assessments within _____. (Agency time frame)

*Job Knowledge*
- Performs wound debridement according to agency protocol.
- Scores Satisfactory on the OASIS instructions test.

## CONCEPT APPLICATION:

### Basing Performance Indicators on Standards of Care *(continued)*

**Home Health Aide**

*Quality*
- Consistently performs skin care according to HHA assignment.
- Uses appropriate positioning and transfer techniques to prevent shear and friction injuries.

*Quantity*
- Consistently reports reddened areas of non-blanching skin over bony prominences on same day recognized.

*Job Knowledge*
- Achieves adequate pressure reduction in a variety of patient settings.
- Recognizes redness and non-blanching areas over bony prominences.
- Demonstrates appropriate positioning and transfer techniques that reduce skin breakdown and friction.

## Guiding Questions

- Are appraisal indicators written objectively?
- Do performance appraisals of all disciplines include important aspects of outcome-based patient care delivery?
- Is the number of indicators manageable? Too numerous?
- Is each indicator essential?
- Do we want to include a single, overall competency measurement or a few essential competencies of particular importance in the appraisal?
- Do managerial and leadership performance appraisals reflect how well these individuals contribute to overall agency outcomes and results?

**3**B

## CONCEPT APPLICATION:
### Identifying Outcome-Based Performance Indicators

Identify which performance appraisal indicators are outcome-based by placing an O-B in the corresponding blank.

_____ 1. Manages pain to the patient or caretaker's level of satisfaction.

_____ 2. Has no patient or caretaker complaints.

_____ 3. Displays initiative in care pathway development.

_____ 4. Uses agency approved patient teaching materials for all patients on care pathways.

_____ 5. Measures all patient outcomes according to policy timeframes.

_____ 6. Offers assistance to co-workers when possible.

_____ 7. Performs appropriate follow-up as indicated for all patient risk assessments performed.

_____ 8. Initiates and manages parenteral infusions without adverse results.

_____ 9. Achieves a score of *Satisfactory* in wound management competency.

_____ 10. Manages pain adequately.

*Answers: 1, 2, 4, 5, 7, 8, & 9*
*Rationale: Statements are measurable and can affect healthcare outcomes.*

## AGENCY APPLICATION:
### Writing Performance Indicators

An agency has experienced less than desired OASIS outcomes for urinary incontinence over a one-year period. It now ranks as the agency's second highest outcome needing remediation and is consistently below the national benchmark, quarter-to-quarter. The agency also has a high incidence of urinary tract infection (UTI) according to infection control reports and the OBQI Adverse Event Outcome report. In the past, the agency performed usual care according to physician orders.

Agency managers decide to implement a care pathway for Urinary Incontinence. After researching best practices, the managers include the following interventions in the pathway:

- Early recognition of untoward signs & symptoms of UTI
- Skin care and moisture control protocol
- Scheduled fluid intake
- Pelvic muscle exercises
- Bladder training
- Prompted voiding
- Use of voiding record
- Medication management

Agency managers decide to include some elements of this standard in their upcoming revision of their performance appraisals.

For each discipline, as appropriate,

1. Prioritize the type and numbers of indicators to include in the revision that will help outline staff responsibilities in improving the agency's outcome of urinary incontinence.
2. Give your rationale for the indicators you write.

**Nurses**

RN_____

_____

_____

LPN_____

_____

_____

**3**B

## AGENCY APPLICATION:
### Writing Performance Indicators *(continued)*

**Therapists**

RPT _____

_____

_____

OT _____

_____

_____

SLP _____

_____

_____

Home Health Aide _____

_____

_____

Social Service _____

_____

_____

## REFERENCES

Beaumont, P. B. (1993). *Human resource management: Key concepts and skills.* Thousand Oaks, CA: Sage Publications.

Capko, J. (2003). Five steps to a performance evaluation system: Keep your staff productive and motivated by conducting regular performance evaluations. *Family Practice Management,* 10(3), 43. Retrieved September 4, 2003 from Infotrac database.

Herringer, J. M. (2002). Once isn't enough when measuring staff competence. *Nursing Management,* 33(2), 22.

McAdams. C. C. & Montgomery, K. A. (2003). Narrowing the possibilities: Using quality improvement tools to decrease competence assessment overload. *Journal for Nurses in Staff Development,* 19(1), 40–46.

Wiles, L. L. & Bishop, J. F. (2001). Clinical performance appraisal: Renewing graded experiences. *Journal of Nursing Education,* 40(1), 37–39.

# Financial Outcomes Data: Use and Application

*Contributed by Colleen Miller, RN, CCRN*

## LEARNING OBJECTIVES

Upon completion of this topic, you will be able to:

1. Evaluate the following financial outcomes relative to outcome-based patient care and agency goals:
   - Average reimbursement (HHRG)
   - Average visits by discipline
   - Average costs by discipline
   - Average supply costs per diagnosis
2. Identify the financial impact of using best practice interventions developed from a clinical practice guideline.
3. Identify clinical assessments and interventions that impact agency financial outcomes.

## AGENCY-SPECIFIC DATA/RESOURCES NEEDED

Top ten diagnoses by admission volume over the last 12 months from Chapter 2, Section A

---

**CORE TERMS AND CONCEPTS**

- Average Reimbursement
- HHRG
- Case mix
- Cost of Care by Discipline
- Supply Costs

# INTRODUCTION

The prospective payment system of reimbursement for homecare providers values the most effective care at the least possible cost (Sienkiewicz and Narayan, 2002). This prompts an agency to continually search for ways to reduce costs while maintaining quality and profitability. Financial outcomes are directly linked to the agency's clinical operations; now more than ever before, they require knowledge of financial and clinical outcomes data to operate effectively (Micheletti, Shlala and Goodall, 1998).

Home care demands more than just claim form/billing data from IS in order to survive in this new environment (Lapin, 2001). Additionally, McCann (2001) recommends a review of agency outcomes and utilization data to manage most efficiently. Administrators must be able to correlate data as they relate to costs, quality of care, resource utilization, and clinical outcomes to drive process improvement as well as revenue. Only then can care quality be improved and costs be controlled.

This chapter describes how to identify, evaluate, and monitor the agency's financial outcomes as related to agency reimbursement, diagnosis, discipline utilization, supply utilization, and cost of care delivery. Cost saving initiatives based on clinical and financial data correlation as well as the financial impact of implementing standards developed from clinical practice guidelines are explored.

Financial outcomes that you calculate in Table 4.1 Agency Application are subsequently carried over to applications that follow. This *building block* approach continues until a set of your agency's financial outcomes are produced in the end for comprehensive analysis.

## IDENTIFYING BASELINE FINANCIAL OUTCOMES

There are six primary financial outcomes that your agency must review on a regular basis. These outcomes keep you abreast of costs of care that can be correlated with clinical outcomes. These are:

- average reimbursement
- average visits by discipline
- average visit costs by discipline
- average discipline costs by diagnosis
- supply utilization
- wound management costs

### Average Reimbursement

Under PPS, reimbursement for the patient's episode is determined by a combination of three factors. An agency receives a *standardized payment* for each Medicare patient's episode of care. This standardized payment is *adjusted* based on the patient's geographic location (wage index) and health status at admission (case mix) (Sienkiewicz and Narayan, 2002). The case mix is based on *responses for 23 specific OASIS data set items*. When the OASIS assessment is complete, responses from the 23 items are added to give Clinical (C), Functional (F), and Service (S) scores for the patient.

Each of these scores is grouped to categorize the patient into a single C-F-S group, also known as a Home Health Resource Group (HHRG). There are 80 HHRGs. Each of the 80 HHRGs has a weighted number (case weight) attached that reflects the intensity of care and cost of care a patient will require (Sienkiewicz and Narayan, 2002). The weighted number is then multiplied by the standardized payment rate for home care to determine the actual reimbursement for a patient's 60-day episode of care (CMS, 2000). The *variety of case weights* of your agency's patients makes up your agency's case mix.

Understanding your case mix provides valuable information, such as the type of patients you are caring for, the average case mix per diagnosis, and average length of stay (LOS) for specific diagnosis groups (Peterson, 2001). This information helps to determine services to add or delete, review staff skill mix, analyze discipline utilization and patient education needs, and identify the acuity level of your patients. For these reasons, you should frequently review your case mix to identify changes in your patient populations.

## AGENCY APPLICATION:
## Average Reimbursement and Case Mix by Diagnosis

A composite HHRG score per diagnosis gives you valuable information that case mix alone cannot give. It provides a quick glance of the intensity of care reflected in each group. For example, if the agency's case mix for CHF is high, the composite quickly reveals which scores contribute to this.

1. In the following table, enter the agency's top ten diagnoses or ICD-9 codes, respective of composite HHRG scores, average case mix (your business office should be able to provide), and corresponding average reimbursement for the last six months, with and without therapy.

2. To obtain a composite HHRG score:

   a) Total a sample of C scores for one diagnosis for an episode of care.
   b) Calculate the average.
   c) Calculate the average for F scores and S scores respectively.

**Table 4.1**  Average Reimbursement and Case Mix

| Diagnosis | Composite HHRG Score C_F_S_ | Average Case Mix | Average Reimbursement with Therapy | Average Reimbursement without Therapy | Total Average Reimbursement with and without Therapy |
|---|---|---|---|---|---|
| Example: 707 | C2F1S0 | 0.8758 | $4,700.00 | $3,000.00 | $3,850.00 |
| 1. | | | | | |
| 2. | | | | | |
| 3. | | | | | |
| 4. | | | | | |
| 5. | | | | | |
| 6. | | | | | |
| 7. | | | | | |
| 8. | | | | | |
| 9. | | | | | |
| 10. | | | | | |

4

Examine your HHRG assignments and case mix in relation to your reimbursement dollars. Look for discrepancies in the HHRG and the acuity of the patient. For example, you know a patient requires a high intensity of service, yet the HHRG assignment and subsequent reimbursement do not reflect this. This should prompt a review of how OASIS assessments are completed by staff, as well as how ICD-9 codes are assigned. The best way to ensure appropriate reimbursement is to ensure that an accurate OASIS assessment is completed and that appropriate ICD-9 coding principles are used (Doughty, M., 2001).

## Average Visits by Discipline

While case weight forms the basis of your reimbursement, managing your resources (visits per episode, discipline utilization, and associated costs) is imperative for your survival (Rooney and Lang, 2003). You want to analyze your visit data by diagnosis. This includes the number of visits by discipline per episode in relation to the HHRG assignment. This analysis identifies problems with visit and discipline utilization.

For example, a patient has S2 or S3 in the HHRG score, but therapy is not scheduled, or therapy has made few visits in the episode, and nursing likewise has few visits scheduled or completed. This has the potential to affect quality of care, as well as the clinical and financial outcomes for both the patient and the agency.

Visit data can identify questionable visit patterns by discipline for the same diagnosis (Lapin, 2001). For example, when reviewing average visits by discipline, you notice that physical therapy makes an average of 12 to 15 visits for each CHF patient, yet nursing makes an average of eight. From reviewing a national benchmark for average case mix, you question the number of visits being made by therapy for this diagnosis.

Verify visit utilization and appropriateness by reviewing the clinical note, the patient's condition, and staff interview. Understanding these patterns and why they occur can also assist you in identifying staff education and competency needs and in building consistent visit utilization by diagnosis.

---

### AGENCY APPLICATION:
### Average Visits by Discipline per Diagnosis

1. From *Table 4.1*, transfer the diagnoses and HHRG data to the following table, *4.2*.

2. For each of the top ten diagnoses identified in *Table 4.1*, calculate the agency's average visits by discipline for an episode of care in the last six months. (Your business office should be able to provide you with this information.)

3. Total the visits performed by each discipline.

4. Divide this figure by the number of staff providing care in each discipline to give you the average visits by discipline.

5. Total the average visits of all disciplines for each diagnosis.

## AGENCY APPLICATION:
### Average Visits by Discipline per Diagnosis *(continued)*

**Table 4.2**  Average Visits/Discipline

| Diagnosis | Average HHRG Score C_ F_ S_ | RN | LPN | PT | OT | ST | MSS | Aide | Total Visits (all disciplines) |
|---|---|---|---|---|---|---|---|---|---|
| *Example: 707.0* | *C2F1S0* | *24* | *0* | *2* | *0* | *0* | *0* | *4* | *30* |
| 1. | | | | | | | | | |
| 2. | | | | | | | | | |
| 3. | | | | | | | | | |
| 4. | | | | | | | | | |
| 5. | | | | | | | | | |
| 6. | | | | | | | | | |
| 7. | | | | | | | | | |
| 8. | | | | | | | | | |
| 9. | | | | | | | | | |
| 10. | | | | | | | | | |

*Guiding Questions*

- Are the visits performed appropriate in relation to the acuity?
- Are the appropriate disciplines caring for the patient?
- What discipline is driving the plan of care (POC)? *(The discipline driving the plan of care typically requires more visits than others.)*
- How does your agency actively monitor visits per discipline per episode, per diagnosis?
- What are the Clinical, Functional, and Service scores in relation to visits per discipline?

4

## Average Visit Costs per Discipline

To identify financial outcomes, determine your agency's costs of care delivery for various patient populations. This includes *individual discipline visit costs* (visit rate and/or salary costs, benefits, and travel (mileage) as well as *total discipline cost per diagnosis*.

## AGENCY APPLICATION:
### Average Visit Costs per Discipline

1. Add your visit costs (agency's visit rate and/or cost of salaries plus benefits and mileage) for each discipline.

2. Divide your total visit costs per discipline by the total number of visits for each discipline.

In the following table, enter your agency's average visit costs per discipline.

**Table 4.3** Average Visit Costs by Discipline

| Discipline | Sample: Average Costs Per Discipline | Your Average Visit Costs Per Discipline |
|---|---|---|
| RN | $90 | |
| LPN | | |
| PT | $100 | |
| OT | | |
| ST | | |
| MSW | | |
| Aide | $35 | |

## Average Discipline Costs by Diagnosis

Evaluate your visit costs per discipline in relation to your reimbursement by diagnosis. From this information you can quickly ascertain your average costs for visiting staff by diagnosis. Be alert to costs that appear disproportionate to reimbursement. Review these findings.

## AGENCY APPLICATION:
### Discipline Costs by Diagnosis

1. From Table 4.1, enter your top ten diagnoses and average reimbursement per discipline to the following Table 4.4.

2. To calculate your average visit costs per discipline per diagnosis:

   a. Multiply the number of visits performed by each discipline for each diagnosis from Table 4.2 by the average visit costs per discipline from Table 4.3.

   b. Enter these figures in their respective columns below.

3. Total all discipline visit costs for each diagnosis and enter in the last column: Total discipline costs.

**Table 4.4** Discipline Costs by Diagnosis

| Diagnosis | Average reimbursement | Average visit costs RN | Average visit costs LPN | Average visit costs PT | Average visit costs OT | Average visit costs SLP | Average visit costs Aide | Average visit costs MSS | Total discipline costs |
|---|---|---|---|---|---|---|---|---|---|
| Example: 707.0 | $3,850 | $2,160 | 0 | $200 | 0 | 0 | $35 | 0 | $2,500 |
| 1. | | | | | | | | | |
| 2. | | | | | | | | | |
| 3. | | | | | | | | | |
| 4. | | | | | | | | | |
| 5. | | | | | | | | | |
| 6. | | | | | | | | | |
| 7. | | | | | | | | | |
| 8. | | | | | | | | | |
| 9. | | | | | | | | | |
| 10. | | | | | | | | | |

Evaluate your discipline visit costs in relation to your reimbursement by diagnosis to get an idea of where your patient populations fall within cost and revenue.

4

## Supply Utilization and Associated Costs

In PPS, the homecare provider has financial responsibility for the patient's medically necessary supplies during the LOS. Medical supplies are items, due to their therapeutic or diagnostic characteristics, essential to effectively perform the care the physician has ordered for the treatment or diagnosis of the patient's illness or injury. Exceptions are those supplies billed separately to Medicare under the Part B Benefit (Sienkiewicz and Narayan, 2002). These include:

- Durable medical equipment (DME) such as walkers or bedside commodes
- Diabetes supplies, when a patient is independent with his or her diabetes management
- Enteral feeding supplies
- Infusion supplies
- Underpads and diapers (unless the POC specifies these items as pertinent to the care the clinicians are providing to the patient)
- Supplies already being provided by the Veterans Administration, unless the patient chooses to have you supply them. The patient must be allowed to choose if he or she would like home care to provide supplies (Sienkiewicz and Narayan, 2002).

In order to gain fiscal control of supply costs, agency management must gain insight into its product lines, product costs, utilization (Barrera, 2002), and clinical outcomes related to specific supply categories, such as wound and diabetic supplies. Macinnes (2002) describes five red flags related to medical supply utilization in home care:

1. Identifying the top five supplies used within the agency and scrutinizing for appropriate use and cost
2. Assessing the utilization and dollars spent by product category
3. Evaluating wound care patient costs and the progress/outcomes between saline and other types of wound care treatment
4. Examining and improving an agency's formulary, monitoring its use and performance, and instituting the practice of direct substitution for *like items*
5. Reviewing monthly purchases over a three-month period; sort from the highest to the lowest level of use. (This information identifies unnecessary and/or duplicated items and associated costs *and* also provides potential opportunities for better pricing contracts for certain high volume products.)

As you begin to evaluate products, and supply inventory and use, examine *total cost* to provide care versus *individual supply item costs* (Ovington, 2001). Do not assume that a less expensive supply item automatically saves dollars overall. A cheaper item may actually cost the agency more if it is associated with an increased incidence of infection or if it creates an obstacle for patient self-management; both of which are undesirable patient outcomes.

## AGENCY APPLICATION:
## Determining Supply Costs

Determine your supply cost by diagnoses.

1. Review the supply use by patients in your top ten diagnoses for an episode of care during the last six months.

2. Calculate your supply costs per patient by diagnosis.

3. Total the supply costs for all patients in each diagnosis.

4. Divide supply costs by number of patients having each diagnosis.

In the following table, enter the supply costs for each diagnosis.

**Table 4.5** Supply Costs for Top Ten Diagnoses

| Diagnosis | Average Supply Costs |
|---|---|
| *Example: 707.0* | *$96.00* |
| 1. | |
| 2. | |
| 3. | |
| 4. | |
| 5. | |
| 6. | |
| 7. | |
| 8. | |
| 9. | |
| 10. | |

You have compiled key information to assist you in managing resources that impact both financial and clinical outcomes. With the amount of data available to home care from both internal and external sources, it is imperative that you determine what data are relevant and how to maximize their use. The true value of data is in their end use, not in their existence (Sblendorio, 2003). Data become valuable when they provide you with insights into the reason for trends, and how your own agency's operation style impacts the trends, as well as the correlation between the trends and your clinical and financial outcomes.

When data work for you to improve your operations and outcomes, you have succeeded in information management. Sblendorio (2003) identifies what executives seek to identify through their data. They include:

- What the organization does or does not do that positively or negatively affects outcomes achievement
- Where the most efficient use of resources (costs) yields the highest clinical outcomes
- Where the highest outcomes occur with a minimum number of encounters using specific care protocols for specific groups of patients

This information provides insight not only to manage your business, but shows how to *strategically* manage your business (Sblendorio, 2003).

Because controlling supply costs, especially wound care supplies, has been one of home care's greatest challenges in the PPS environment (Doughty, D., 2001), wound management and its supplies deserves a closer examination. This text uses its basis for moist wound healing from AHRQ's clinical practice guideline for the treatment of pressure ulcers (DHHS, 2000). *Moist wound healing* is defined as tissues remaining moist during the healing process. *Advanced wound dressing* refers to dressings that have been designed to be moisture retentive such as polyurethane films, foams, hydrogels, and hydrocolloids, as well as calcium alginates and collagens (Kwon, 2001; Ovington, 2001).

## Managing Costs Related to Wound Care

Over the last 25 to 30 years, wound products have evolved into high-tech applications. As manufacturers began to understand the concept of *moist wound healing*, they began to develop dressings to maintain moisture and to prevent wound desiccation (Ovington, 2001). There are now literally hundreds of products available for wound management.

Sorting through different types of products and their effective and efficient use, while controlling costs and achieving positive clinical outcomes, continues to present a challenge. You may require assistance from a Wound Ostomy Continence Nurse (WOCN) or wound specialist to determine the products or product line(s) that are cost-effective and best meet the needs of your patients.

Cost of products and labor costs for product use should be examined when considering products for agency inventory. It is imperative that administrators consider all costs associated with the delivery of wound care prior to selecting the agency's product inventory and building a wound care formulary. According to Dr. Liza Ovington (2001), the *real cost* of wound care can be considered as:

- the price of the dressing, plus
- the labor cost of having a healthcare professional change the dressing, plus
- the indirect costs of ancillary supplies and services used in changing the dressings (e.g., gloves and biohazardous waste disposal), plus
- the cost of the duration of care (e.g., facility charges and travel costs for homecare nurses).

Note that a *true* total cost of care also includes patient outcomes achieved. A dressing that costs less may actually cost the agency more if positive patient outcomes are not attained. You may calculate your supply costs two ways. One way is to add all supplies used for all patients for each diagnosis for a specific period of time to give you supply costs per diagnosis. The second is to determine if your business office has a dollar amount (a percent of charges) that is applied to each patient for nonroutine supplies use when calculating direct costs.

## AGENCY APPLICATION:
### Calculating Wound Supply Costs

1. Examine the supply costs for a 60 day episode of care for a patient with a stage 3 or 4 pressure ulcer.

2. Enter each supply item used for wound care and its cost.

3. Determine the quantity of each supply item used during the 60 day episode of care.

4. Multiply the quantity of each supply item by the individual cost of the supply item (unit price) to obtain the *total cost per item*.

5. Add totals to give you the cost of supplies for a 60 day episode of care.

**Table 4.6**  Example: 1000 4x4s used at a cost of ten cents each =
1000 x .10 = $100

| Supply Item(s) | Quantity Used Per Episode | X | Unit Price | = | Total Cost Per Item |
|---|---|---|---|---|---|
| 4x4 | 1000 | | .10 | | $100 |
| 2x2 | 700 | | .05 | | $35 |
| | | | | Total supply costs: | $135 |

**Table 4.7**  Calculating Wound Supply Costs

Pressure Ulcer: Stage _____

| Supply Item(s) | Quantity Used Per Episode | X | Unit Price | = | Total Cost Per Item |
|---|---|---|---|---|---|
| | | | | | |
| | | | | | |
| | | | | | |
| | | | | | |
| | | | | Total wound supply cost(s) per episode: $ | |

4

## AGENCY APPLICATION:
### Direct Costs of Providing Wound Care

Direct costs are defined as *the cost of care attributed to hands-on care in the home* (Hagenow, 1999). Determine your agency's direct costs of providing care to a patient with a stage 3 or 4 pressure ulcer for a 60 day episode of care. In the following table, enter the data from your pressure ulcer patients for supply costs; enter *actual supply costs per patient* or the dollar amount (multiplied by the number of patients in each diagnosis) that is reflective of a percent of charges obtained from your business office. Add your discipline visit costs to your supply costs to obtain your direct costs for your pressure ulcer patient.

**Table 4.8** Direct Costs of Pressure Ulcer Care

| Diagnosis | Average Reimbursement | Total Visits by Discipline | Total Discipline Visit Costs | Average Wound Supply Costs | Total Direct Cost of Wound Care |
|---|---|---|---|---|---|
| *Pressure Ulcer* | | | | | |

## CONCEPT APPLICATION:
## Comparing Costs of Wound Treatment Modalities

Compare the cost differences in treatment plans using traditional saline and gauze dressings versus best practice of moist wound dressings for a stage 3 pressure ulcer. The example in Table 4.9 reveals total costs of a traditional modality for wound treatment, while Table 4.10 shows the costs of advanced dressings associated with moist wound healing, recommended from a clinical practice guideline.

**Table 4.9**  Example: Traditional Saline and Gauze (Wet-to-Dry)
(Pressure Ulcer Stage 3 without Therapy)

| | | | |
|---|---|---|---|
| Avg. reimbursement for Stage 3 pressure ulcer = | | **$3,000** | Per 60-day episode |
| Avg. visit frequency | BID = | 14 vs./wk = | 120 vs./episode |
| Avg. cost per discipline | RN | $90/vs. = | $10,800 (90x120) |
| Avg. supply costs | Wet-to-dry with saline | **$3 per dressing change =** | **$360 (3x120)** |
| Supplies included:<br>Dressing<br>Gloves<br>Irrigation syringe<br>Saline<br>Tape | | **Total Cost =** | **$12,160** |

**Table 4.10**  Example: Use of AHRQ or WOCN Clinical Practice Guideline of Moist Wound Healing (Pressure Ulcer Stage 3 without Therapy)

| | | | |
|---|---|---|---|
| Avg. reimbursement for Stage 3 pressure ulcer = | | **$3,000** | Per 60-day episode |
| Avg. visit frequency | 3 vs./wk = | 3 vs./wk = | 24 vs./episode |
| Avg. cost per discipline | RN | $90/vs. = | $2,160 (90x24) |
| Avg. supply costs | Advanced dressing | **$12 per dressing change =** | **$288 (12x24)** |
| | | **Total Cost =** | **$2,458** |

Moist wound healing decreases the total cost of care secondary to the longevity of the dressing; the time between dressing changes is decreased, thereby decreasing the number of skilled visits required (Ovington, 2001). Note that even though actual dressing costs are higher, the number of visits required to change the dressing is much less, thus decreasing the total cost of this wound treatment.

*Guiding Questions*

- What is the agency's current use of clinical practice guidelines for wound care?
- What is your staff's knowledge regarding wound clinical practice guidelines?

- Do you have access to a WOCN or wound specialty nurse for consultation and staff development?
- Who is responsible for the cost-effectiveness of supplies and use?
- Is supply stock organized by product category for efficient use? If not, who will be responsible to make this happen?
- Does the agency have supply contracts that provide for better pricing? If not, who can assume this responsibility?

At this point you are probably thinking the supplies we use are those that are ordered by the patient's physician. This is true. However, are the outcomes achieved what the physician desires? What the agency desires? What the patient and caretaker desire? Benchmark your outcomes by wound type and share this information with your referral sources as it relates to their practice patterns. The following application is an example of how to aggregate practice pattern data to share with referral sources, as you deem appropriate.

---

## AGENCY APPLICATION:

### Evaluating the Agency's Use of Moist Wound Healing versus Traditional Wet-to-Dry Dressings

Determine the percentage of patients who have been treated with traditional wet-to-dry dressings versus advanced wound dressings. Conduct a medical record review of your agency's patients who have received treatment for complicated open surgical wounds and Stage 3 and 4 pressure ulcers over the past six months.

In *Table 4.11*:

- Enter the medical record number.
- Note the physician.
- Enter the average number of episodes and total visits per episode.
- Note whether the dressing used is wet-to-dry, advanced, or a combination.

**Table 4.11** Evaluation of Agency Wound Treatment Modalities

| Medical Record Number | Physician | Average LOS in Episodes | Total Visits Per Episode | Wet-to-Dry Dressing Use Yes or No | Advanced Dressing Yes or No | Combination of Both Yes or No |
|---|---|---|---|---|---|---|
| | | | | | | |
| | | | | | | |
| | | | | | | |
| | | | | | | |
| | | | | | | |
| | | | | | | |

---

Using this information, evaluate the types of dressings used in your agency. Using your agency's costs and reimbursement figures from previous applications, how do your agency's financial outcomes for the two wound treatments and costs compare? This information can be powerful because it can have a potentially positive affect on physician practice patterns and ultimately on your patients' clinical outcomes.

For referral sources that have less-than-desired patient outcomes, use this opportunity to discuss your agency's findings, goals for patients, and treatment options. Also, discuss the use of advanced dressings and patient benefits from this treatment modality, as well as the outcomes documented in the literature. Be prepared to provide current literature on the use of advanced wound dressings. Literature can be obtained from websites *(See Appendix A: Internet Resource Listing: Best Practices)* and from your wound product vendors. As appropriate, request that your referral source allow you one patient for which to use an advanced dressing in place of wet-to-dry. Share the results of both financial and clinical outcomes for that source's *trial* patient.

Thus far we have explored reimbursement, discipline costs, visit costs, supply costs, and product use as they affect the agency's financial outcomes. There is also a financial impact associated with specific clinical assessments and interventions performed routinely by staff.

## THE EFFECT OF CLINICAL ASSESSMENTS AND INTERVENTIONS ON FINANCIAL OUTCOMES

Clinicians make decisions on a daily basis that not only affect clinical patient outcomes, but agency financial outcomes as well. Let's examine how clinical assessment and intervention affects reimbursement and costs by examining the following:

- Accuracy of OASIS documentation
- ICD-9 Coding
- Care Coordination
- Clinician's Use of Supplies

### OASIS Assessment Accuracy

In addition to yielding patient outcomes, the OASIS data set items are designed to determine reimbursement for care according to patient status at the time of the assessment (CMS, 2002). Inaccurately recorded OASIS assessment data can affect case mix and result in the loss of appropriate reimbursement or in over-reimbursement, and can result in invalid clinical outcomes. How do inaccuracies occur?

Clinicians can have a lack of knowledge of OASIS response instructions (CMS, 2002). For example, a clinician who does not know the instructions incorrectly assesses the ability of the patient to *Perform Activities of Daily Living*. An invalid assessment is documented and case mix is negatively affected. If additional items are assessed using incorrect response instructions, reimbursement can be negatively affected by hundreds of dollars and can be inadequate to cover the agency's cost of providing care.

*Guiding Questions*

- Is ongoing OASIS documentation education and training being conducted?
- Is attendance adequate?
- How are skilled staff deemed competent in completing OASIS assessments?

### ICD-9 Coding

The proper coding and coding sequence of diagnoses can also directly affect financial outcomes. For example, improper use of coding principles may result in a clinician entering *Diabetes* as a secondary diagnosis when it should be the primary diagnosis. When this happens, both case mix and reimbursement are negatively affected. As well, coding inaccuracy multiplied by several patients substantially affects overall reimburse-

NOTES

ment. To avoid incorrect coding of diagnoses, individuals responsible for coding must be competent in:

- Current coding principles
- Coding diabetes, neoplasm, and wounds correctly
- Correctly identifying the type of wound and/or the stage of pressure ulcers
- Coding to the 4th and 5th digit of specificity
- Identifying diagnosis codes that provide reimbursement appropriate to the complexity of care
- Proper use of V and E codes
- Proper sequencing of diagnosis codes

It is important that clinicians understand the impact that OASIS assessment and ICD-9 coding have on agency revenue, and the role each clinician plays in the agency's receiving appropriate reimbursement for care provision.

## Guiding Questions

- Are skilled staff or appropriate individuals competent in ICD-9 coding principles?
- Is ongoing coding education being provided by knowledgeable instructors?
- Does the agency need a professional coder to guide proper coding on a daily basis?

## Care Coordination

Care coordination can have beneficial effects on clinical and financial outcomes. From a *clinical perspective*, care coordination affords clinicians and managers the opportunity to collaborate on patients' needs, progress made, prevention of acute complications, and possible emergent care use and acute care admissions, as well as an evaluation of overall quality of care.

From a *financial perspective*, information can be shared regularly regarding LOS, visit utilization per discipline, supply utilization, prevention of duplicate services, and the evaluation of the treatment plan for appropriateness; all of which affect your agency's bottom line.

For example, consider the coordination of discipline utilization. The clinician performing an initial evaluation or follow-up patient assessment frequently makes unilateral decisions regarding visit frequency and duration. Often this decision is made without knowledge of visits being generated by other disciplines. Without coordinating efforts, some visits may result in unnecessary overlap. This can be avoided by coordinating visits and reviewing care interventions from an overall perspective.

In another example, visit coordination and enhanced communication between occupational and physical therapy can avoid many duplicate exercise interventions. Additionally, certain exercise interventions can be delegated to the home health aide, who has been trained and is competent in such tasks. Be creative in developing the right tools and or approaches to ensure communication among all disciplines and managers in the care coordination process.

## Guiding Questions

- Does the agency's care coordination process include a review of interventions by each discipline?
- Is management regularly involved in coordinating this effort? Directing this process?
- Is the overlap of discipline interventions discussed?
- Is task delegation to other disciplines routinely considered as a method of efficient and cost-effective care provision?

## Clinician's Use of Supplies

Supply costs have relevance to visits and LOS (i.e., number of episodes, visits per episode) that must not be overlooked. As a patient's condition improves, you expect the acuity, as well as reimbursement, to decrease. It is also logical that the visit and supply utilization will decrease with each subsequent episode. Ensure the desired patient outcome and the agency's financial goals by staying abreast of patient progress and monitoring visit utilization and supply costs per episode.

To help control utilization of wound supplies and associated costs, develop a wound care formulary. If you are using like products from multiple vendors, decrease options to one or two like products through specific vendors and secure product contracts to receive better pricing. Develop standardized wound care management strategies and care protocols for your wound population (Flow, 2001) to help you identify certain product types necessary for your inventory.

Begin to review supplies/product lines and utilization by conducting a complete inventory of what is presently in supply room stock. It is imperative that your inventory be based on your primary patient population(s). Physician preference does impact this decision greatly and cannot be ignored. However, basing your inventory on physician or staff preference alone is opening the door to uncontrollable expense. Educate your staff on appropriateness and utilization of supplies and products. Sharing clinical and financial outcomes data with your staff, physicians, and other referral sources is a good place to begin affecting their use of supplies.

## Clinician's Use of Best Practice Interventions

In addition to having a positive impact on patient outcomes, implementing best practice interventions can positively impact costs and financial outcomes (Potts and Jarvis, 2001). You have seen this demonstrated in the comparison of two types of wound dressings. Other interventions can also have an impact on costs.

For example, an agency provides glucometers for its skilled nurses to use when patients do not have their own. One glucometer requires test strips that cost more, but the device prompts more timely calibration than others. Agency managers determine that the intervention of timely calibration promotes safe and proper treatment, and the glucometer with more expensive test strips is chosen. This agency's clinical outcome of timeliness with calibration is good; however, the cost to achieve this is higher. A second agency conducts a thorough search of product lines and locates a glucometer that achieves both goals: timely calibration and less expense overall. This agency's clinical and financial outcomes are both positively affected.

In another example, Agency A is the only one in a local area that provides diapers by the bag for patients with urinary incontinence. Administration believes this to be an important customer service gesture, even though the supply costs are high. The agency provides usual care that does not routinely include bladder training, timed voiding, and special diet and fluid considerations. Its OASIS outcome of urinary incontinence is higher than the national benchmark average.

The agency's competitor provides diapers only during visits when care is provided. However, the competitor implements a urinary incontinence program on admission. All skilled nurses are knowledgeable in its interventions and in its application. The agency markets this approach by promoting the program to physician customers and patients alike. The agency's OASIS outcome of *urinary incontinence* is significantly less than the national benchmark average and its supply costs are less than Agency A.

4

**Table 4.12** Quick Glance Summary: How the Clinician Affects Agency Financials

| Clinical Assessment & Intervention | Questions to Ask | Financial Impact |
| --- | --- | --- |
| OASIS documentation | Is it accurate and complete? | Impact on reimbursement |
| ICD-9 coding | Are coding principles used? Is coding documented correctly? | Impact on reimbursement |
| Care coordination (all disciplines) | Is it occurring regularly? | Impact on cost to agency |
| Supplies: type and utilization | Are supplies appropriate and use consistent among staff? | Impact on cost to agency |
| Best practice interventions | Has implementation occurred and is utilization consistent? | Impact on cost to agency |

## ANALYZING FINANCIAL OUTCOMES DATA OF SPECIFIC POPULATIONS

It is important to know your discipline costs in relation to your reimbursement for each patient population you serve (Peterson, 2001). You must be able to identify where your patient populations fit in relation to cost and revenue (Potts, 2001). For example, what patient population(s) fall into the optimal category of high revenue/low cost? What patient populations are high revenue/high costs, low revenue/ low cost, low revenue/high cost? Determine the interventions needed to maximize revenue and explore cost saving initiatives. For example, for your high revenue/high cost diagnoses, isolate the origin of costs and determine how care can be more cost-efficient. Your investigation and subsequent activities may help this patient population move into the high revenue/low cost category.

Another example: your wound care patients have high costs when compared to a published national average. What is the cause? Is supply usage controlled adequately? Are there too many wound products in your inventory? Are nurses and patients using products efficiently? When evaluating therapy utilization, is there an increased use of therapy without the substantiation of OASIS documentation?

In another example, consider costs of patient care guided by a care pathway. Look at the average reimbursement per episode for the pathway diagnosis and the average visits per discipline. Estimate your average direct visit cost that will be generated from the pathway. (Include salaries, mileage, and supply use.) Also consider direct management cost, if any, involved in using the pathway on a day-to-day basis. Some agencies may have managers who make visits on a weekly basis or who will be highly involved in managing the patient on a pathway.

## CONCEPT APPLICATION:
### Financial Data Analysis

Organizing financial outcomes data in a spreadsheet or table provides for easy evaluation, comparison, and correlation. Examine the following example spreadsheet containing patient financial outcomes data for a 60 day episode of care. Profit (loss) has been included.

**Profit (Loss) = Reimbursement minus (Total Visit Costs + Supply Costs).**

The data below are based on a completed OASIS assessment and plan of care. Based on the data given, what problems can you identify that need investigation and follow-up?

**Figure 4.13** Example: Financial Data Analysis

| Diagnosis | HHRG | Average Case Mix | Reimbursement | Visits per discipline (nursing, therapy, aides) | Total visit costs (nursing, therapy, aides) | Supply Costs | Profit (Loss) |
|---|---|---|---|---|---|---|---|
| Decubitus (707) | C1F2S0 | 0.8758 | $2,700 | N-21 PT-2 HHA-4 | $2,190 | $63 | $447 |

## Guiding Questions

- Is the diagnosis of decubitus (ICD-9 code 707) specific enough?
- With an F2 in the HHRG assignment, why have only two therapy visits been scheduled or ordered?
- Is the case mix accurately depicting the intensity of service for the patient?
- Is the OASIS assessment accurate?

4

## AGENCY APPLICATION:
### Financial Outcomes Analyses by Agency Diagnosis

1. In the following table, enter the financial outcomes for your top ten diagnoses. This information combines all patients with and without therapy.
   *Note: You may choose to separate your data to view profit and loss by diagnosis with and without therapy.*

2. Obtain your top diagnoses, HHRG, case mix, and total average reimbursement from Table 4.1.

3. Obtain visits per discipline per diagnosis from Table 4.2, and discipline visit costs per diagnosis from Table 4.4.

4. Obtain your supply cost per diagnosis from Table 4.10.

5. Evaluate the profit (loss) of each diagnosis by subtracting your discipline and supply costs from your reimbursement for each diagnosis.

**Table 4.14** Agency Financial Outcomes Analysis

| Diagnosis | Average HHRG | Average Case Mix | Average Reimbursement with and without Therapy | Total Discipline Visits (Nursing, Therapy, Aides) | Total Discipline Visit Costs (Nursing, Therapy, Aides) | Average Supply Costs per Discipline | Profit (Loss) |
|---|---|---|---|---|---|---|---|
| Example: 707.0 | C2F1S0 | 0.8758 | $3,850 | 30 | $2,500 | $96 | $1,254 |
|  |  |  |  |  |  |  |  |
|  |  |  |  |  |  |  |  |
|  |  |  |  |  |  |  |  |
|  |  |  |  |  |  |  |  |
|  |  |  |  |  |  |  |  |
|  |  |  |  |  |  |  |  |
|  |  |  |  |  |  |  |  |
|  |  |  |  |  |  |  |  |
|  |  |  |  |  |  |  |  |
|  |  |  |  |  |  |  |  |

### Guiding Questions

Based on the previous data, determine the following:

- Which diagnoses appear to generate an adequate reimbursement in relation to your costs?
- Which diagnoses cost the most to treat? What are generating these costs?
- What interventions can be instituted to maximize revenue and/or control costs?

# FINANCIAL OUTCOME REPORTS

As you have seen throughout this chapter, financial outcomes data can be organized in a variety of ways to assist you in data evaluation and analysis. You can separate these data into basic categories for evaluation by the agency manager or you can view multiple data elements in a spreadsheet to see the agency's overall financial outcomes picture.

For example, you may want to evaluate patterns of resource utilization per diagnosis in relation to your average case mix only. Or, you may want to isolate your most profitable diagnosis groups to examine the case mix, reimbursement, and resource utilization for each diagnosis. Once you have isolated the data you need to impact positive financial outcomes, your software system should enable you to report the data you want.

Talk with your IS staff to discuss the financial data you need and how you need the information organized. Assist them in building reports that generate useful information. If you do not have IS staff, consider purchasing or leasing software that meets your financial outcomes data and reporting needs, and that integrates well with your agency's current database.

## Guiding Questions

- Is IS expertise available to help build the financial outcome reports that we need?
- What types of financial outcomes data are we capable of generating?
- Who needs these data on an agency operational level?
- What types of financial data can we generate by hand, if necessary?
- Who will generate these data on a periodic basis?

## REFERENCES

Barrera, R. (2002). Six key ways to look at cost reduction. *Remington Report*, 10(6) 6, 8–9.

Centers for Medicare and Medicaid Services, U.S. Department of Health and Human Services. (2000). Medicare program prospective payment system for home health agencies: Final rule. *Federal Register*, 65(128), 41128–41214. Retrieved October 9, 2003 from http://www.gpoaccess.gov/fr/retrieve.html.

Centers for Medicare and Medicaid Services, U.S. Department of Health and Human Services. (2002). Outcome-based quality improvement (OBQI) implementation manual.

Doughty, D. (2001). Accurate documentation of wound status under the OASIS system: Standardize the language of wound care. *Remington Report*, 9(5), 26. Retrieved September 12, 2003 from http://www.remingtonreport.com/cart.asp?article_ID=112.

Doughty, M. (2001). Applying ICD-9 CM coding guidelines in home care. *Remington Report*, 9(1), 14. Retrieved September 12, 2003 from http://www.remingtonreport.com/cart.asp?article_ID=5.

Flow, S. (2001). Continuum of care: Wound programs save $43,600 in medical supply expenses and create successful physician relations. *Remington Report*, 9(16), 18. Retrieved September 12, 2003 from http://www.remingtonreport.com/cart.asp?article_ID=102.

Hagenow, N. R. (1999). Examining the dollars and cents of care. *Nursing Management*, 30(3). Retrieved October 9, 2003 from http://www.nursingcenter.com/prodev/ce_article.asp?tid=236506.

Kwon, L. S. (2001). A doctor's perspective on moist wound healing. *Remington Report*, 9(3), 66. Retrieved April 24, 2003 from http://www.remingtonreport.com/cart.asp?article_ID=86.

Lapin, L. M. (2001). Data management: Strategies to bridge financial & clinical information. *Remington Report*, 9(6), 34.

Macinnes, S. (2002). The red flag: Medical supply utilization—5 ways to increase profitability. *Remington Report*, 10(4), 4.

McCann, B. (2001). Mining oasis data to demonstrate the value of your agency and of home health care. *Remington Report*, 9(3), 14. Retrieved April 24, 2003 from http://www.remingtonreport.com/cart.asp?article_ID=78.

Micheletti, J. A., Shlala, T. J, & Goodall, C. R. (1998). Evaluating performance outcomes measurement systems: Concerns and considerations. *Journal of Healthcare Quality*. Retrieved January 14, 2003 from http://www.nahq.org/journal/ce/o64/064.htm.

Ovington, L. G. (2001). Hanging wet-to-dry dressings out to dry. *Home Healthcare Nurse*, 19(8), 477.

Peterson, M. (2001). Building a roadmap to analyze and manage information. *Remington Report*, 9(5), 36; 38–40; 42; 44.

Potts, J. (2001). How to harness the power of data. *Remington Report*, 9(3), 76–77.

Potts, J. & Jarvis, D. (2001). A PPS analysis tool: Projecting the financial impact of clinical protocol changes. *The Remington Report*, 9(5), 46–47.

Rooney, H. & Lang, C. (2003). Key performance measures: Benchmark data from more than 5 million records representing more than 1,000 agencies. *Remington Report*, 11(1), 14; 16–18; 20.

Sblendorio, S. (2003). From data overload to information management and decision support. *Remington Report* web quest. Retrieved October 9, 2003 from http://www.remingtonreport.com.

Sienkiewicz, J. & Narayan, M. C. (2002). Have you mastered PPS? *Home Health Nurse*, 20(5), 308–317.

U.S. Department of Health and Human Services. (2000). Clinical practice guideline: Pressure ulcers in adults. Agency for Healthcare Research and Quality. Retrieved August 21, 2003 from http://hstat.nlm.nih.gov/hq/Hquest/db/local.ahcpr.quick.putq/screen.

**4**

# Using Outcomes Data to Enhance Marketing & Business Development

*Contributed by Colleen Miller, RN, CCRN*

## LEARNING OBJECTIVES

Upon completion of this topic, you will able to:

1. Identify competitive strategies to build long-term working relationships.
2. Identify key referral sources and their specific patient populations served.
3. Interpret and use patient outcomes data for sales and marketing activities.
4. Plan and prepare outcomes data for customer presentations.

## AGENCY-SPECIFIC DATA/RESOURCES NEEDED

- Top ten referral sources by volume over the last 12 months
- Physician satisfaction results for the last 12 months
- Characteristics of patients admitted by top referral sources
  - Diagnosis
  - Gender
  - Payer source

---

**CORE TERMS AND CONCEPTS**

- Key referral source
- Patient populations—characteristics and demographics
- Interpreting and marketing clinical outcomes
- Physician practice patterns

# INTRODUCTION

The homecare market is highly competitive, providing many choices for physicians, discharge planners, and managed care organizations (MCOs). You must position yourself as different and unique in what you have to offer your customers (Dinsdale and Taylor, 2003). It is now more important than ever to market and best serve your existing customers (Bly, 2003), while gaining new market share. Implementing an outcome-based care approach is one way to distinguish yourself among other homecare providers by delivering quality, cost-efficient care through best practice interventions, clinical and financial data collection, and outcomes measurement.

The measurement of outcomes to demonstrate the effectiveness of care is essential (Hill, 1999). Increasingly, quality is being emphasized as a key factor in determining from whom and when care should be received (Rich and Davis, 2002). The second, more challenging task, is building competitive strategies to formulate long-term relationships with your referral sources. This involves more than leaving complimentary treats for physicians or hospitals; it requires an effort to ascertain needs and actively strive to meet those needs.

This chapter offers tips in evaluating your key referral sources and identifying their specific needs, as well as identifying strategies that build long-term working relationships. It demonstrates how to evaluate patient characteristics and demographics specific to each key referral source, how to analyze and interpret agency outcomes data for marketing and sales, and how to prepare outcome presentations for customers.

## IDENTIFYING KEY REFERRAL SOURCES AND THEIR NEEDS

Know your *key* or top physicians and be able to meet their needs in order to build physician loyalty and gain market share (Dinsdale and Taylor, 2003). Identify other key referral sources as well. Key referral sources are typically those who:

- Generate a high volume of referrals who are accepted for admission.
- Use home care sparingly, but primarily choose your agency when home care is ordered.
- Call your agency first to provide infusion therapy, because of quality of service, timeliness of response, and coordination of service.

Key referral sources may directly and indirectly affect other referrals you receive. They are physicians, nurse practitioners, hospital and skilled care discharge planners, office specialty nurses, infusion companies, office managers, and managed care staff and medical directors.

Physicians using home care may send patients to a variety of agencies; many times they are not able to recall the names of agencies used, if asked (Ratner, 2002b). This is not conducive to a strong, long-term working relationship that encompasses trust, loyalty, or commitment.

In order to develop a working relationship with your physicians, you must understand what their needs are and what they want out of the relationship (Ratner, 2002b). You must identify the rewards, answer the *what's-in-it-for-me* question, and identify the primary self interests for both the agency and the referral source (Wincel, 2002). Discovering these needs and acting upon the information will make the difference between you and your competitor.

To begin this process, ask your referral sources what their needs are, what they are looking for in a homecare provider. It may be they are most concerned with a high level of customer service. They may be looking for a provider that offers other services in addition to home care such as private duty or hospice. They may have interest in an agency that can provide special clinical skills for certain diagnoses, or quantifiable outcomes data.

Determine what their preferences are for communication with your agency and clinicians. In addition, talk with your staff and elicit feedback about their relationships with your key physicians. Investigate how they presently communicate information, what information they provide, and the timeliness of the exchange.

Review physician satisfaction surveys to determine what they feel you are doing well, and where you have opportunities for improvement. Look for correlations between physician concerns, patient populations served, and agency resources, skill sets, or services. Identify what you are doing now that keeps the top referral sources using your agency services, and what you are doing that sets you apart from the competition. These activities will assist you in laying a foundation for maintaining relationships and building new ones to enhance future growth.

---

### AGENCY APPLICATION:
### Identifying Key Referral Sources and Their Needs

- List your top ten key referral sources, first by admission volume.

- Refine this list by using other criteria of importance to your agency. For example, a referral source may not generate a large volume now, but you may have plans for a new service that involves a particular referral source. Include this source in your list. Also use physician satisfaction surveys, compliments, concerns, or complaints to obtain information.

1._____

2._____

3._____

4._____

5._____

6._____

7._____

8._____

9._____

10. _____

---

## IDENTIFYING POPULATIONS SPECIFIC TO
## KEY REFERRAL SOURCES

Identifying your agency's patient populations is the preface to identifying and analyzing the patient population characteristics of your key referral sources (Potts, 2001). Knowing the types and acuity of patients based on the referral source allows you to better analyze the services and staff skills relative to specific needs of the referral source.

For example, Dr. X admits most of his profitable Medicare patients to another agency, while he admits several nonprofitable patients to you. Aggregated patient characteris-

5

tics give you objective information to analyze this issue. If enhancing agency efficiency and cost-effectiveness for this patient group does not solve this problem, share your quantified data with Dr. X. Do not assume that a physician knows which homecare agency he or she uses the most.

---

### AGENCY APPLICATION:
### Aggregating Statistics for Referral Sources

If your agency does not have software that can aggregate the following information for you, obtain it manually from your records or other reports and perform the calculation.

*From one of your high-volume referral sources*, review and aggregate the following characteristics of a large, representative sample of Medicare patients having the same primary diagnosis:

Average Age:                    F_____    M _____

Gender:                         _____ %Female _____ %Male

Average Reimbursement:          _____

Average Cost of Care Delivery:  _____

Note your findings.

---

## COMPETITIVE STRATEGIES THAT BUILD CUSTOMER RELATIONSHIPS

Despite the challenges, building long-term working relationships with your key referrals is rewarding (Ratner, 2002b). A single primary-care physician with a large number of geriatric or chronically ill patients can generate hundreds of referrals a year. In addition, physician specialists such as a neurologist or endocrinologist may see large numbers of high acuity patients and can provide large number of referrals to home care. As a result, physicians play a key role in cash flow to the agency (Ratner, 2002a).

Investigate ways to customize relationships with key referral sources. These may include:

- Aggregating patient outcomes specific to the patients of a particular referral source. For example, you periodically provide a cardiology group practice with their home care patients' aggregated clinical and financial outcomes relative to the care you are rendering.
- A specific intake access number.
- A simplified, customized referral form that is faxed or e-mailed.
- Periodic education programs for physician staff regarding reimbursement, regulations, and care plan oversight.
- Regular clinical and continuing education offerings for MCO nursing staff
- Creative ways to communicate with physicians that do not compete with their office practice hours.

You can enhance and build long-term customer relations with referral sources in a variety of ways. Wincel (2002) describes four precepts to be cognizant of when building customer relationships:

1. *Accept that competing self-interests are the basis for the customer relationship.* You need referrals to survive, and your referrals need the avenue of home care.
2. *Establish measurable objectives for success based on the identified needs.* These objectives should project the measurable value of the relationship to both parties. Measure quality of care through outcomes, length of stay, referrals per month, or the level of customer service perceived by your customers.
3. *Collaboratively develop products, programs, or processes for mutual success.* This may include staff development initiatives for referral source office staff, developing practice standards or care pathways that meet the needs of your physician's patients, or participating in a disease management initiative to address the needs of high volume/high acuity/high cost patients.
4. *Regularly and objectively evaluate the overall success and value of the relationship.* The success and enduring nature of any relationship is based upon outcomes (Morrow, 2001; Wincel, 2002). Regardless of the type of relationship, offer to aggregate homecare outcomes for patients specific to a referral source. For example, your agency enters into an alliance with the local hospital to establish a continuum of care. You recommend developing a set of mutually agreed upon clinical and financial outcomes. The care pathway reflects interventions that home care will continue post-hospital discharge with the goals being to decrease hospital readmissions and to decrease hospital length of stay.

These outcomes are shared with the hospital on a periodic basis.

---

### AGENCY APPLICATION:
### Building Customer Relationships

List agency initiatives you have implemented that you feel have solidified customer relationships.

_____

_____

_____

_____

List others that have potential for implementation in the future.

_____

_____

_____

_____

---

5

# CLINICAL OUTCOMES DATA FOR MARKETING AND SALES

Experts agree that the homecare industry is on the verge of a significant evolution, one that centers on unprecedented focus on quality management (Rooney and Lang, 2003). One area receiving much attention and concern is the public release of agency-specific outcomes data through *Home Health Compare* by CMS. The key for homecare agencies to survive this aggressive agenda is clear: *Homecare agencies must tell their own story* (Rooney and Lang, 2003). An agency must use this opportunity to strategically position itself by knowing and understanding its own data better than surveyors, payers, physicians, patients, or the public.

To do this, the agency must prioritize information and data from both internal and external sources, and use the data in combination with experience to paint an accurate and credible picture of performance (Rooney and Lang, 2003), quality of care, and financial and clinical outcomes.

Agencies must understand how their outcomes compare to their competitors, as well as to national benchmarks (Sblendorio, 2003). National benchmarks are necessary for self-evaluation and comparison, and for putting your agency's performance in perspective. Thus, for agencies to strategically position themselves in advance of information being made public, they benefit from access to more frequent, real-time data (Lapin, 2001; Rooney and Lang, 2003). One way this can be accomplished is through the development and measurement of agency supplemental outcomes data.

---

## CONCEPT APPLICATION:
### Using Outcomes Data for Marketing and Sales

Your agency receives a large number of wound patients, including those with pressure ulcer(s), from a specific referral source. You have implemented recommended best practice interventions for pressure ulcer care. You have identified patient *outcomes* that are used for measurement and comparison. These are:

*Outcome 1 (OASIS): Emergent care for wound infection, deteriorating wound status*

*Outcome 2 (OASIS): Increase in number of pressure ulcers*

*Outcome 3 (Agency): Patient/caretaker demonstrates appropriate wound care management (i.e., dressing change, wound cleansing)*

*Outcome 4 (Agency): Patient/caretaker verbalizes signs and symptoms of wound infection and/or deterioration; Reports to homecare nurse or physician.*

*Outcome 5 (Agency): Patient/caretaker demonstrates proper pressure relief.*

Outcomes data are extrapolated for the patient population of this referral source for one quarter and are aggregated into percentages.

## CONCEPT APPLICATION:
## Using Outcomes Data for Marketing and Sales *(continued)*

*Example:*

Sample size of pressure ulcer patients: 15

Outcome 1:   1/15 = 6%      (One patient requires emergent care for wound infection/deteriorating wound status)

Outcome 2:   0/15 = 0%      (Zero patients have an increase in pressure ulcers)

Outcome 3:   13/15 = 86%    (Thirteen patients demonstrate wound management)

Outcome 4:   14/15 = 93%    (Fourteen patients verbalize S/S of infection/deterioration)

Outcome 5:   15/15 = 100%   (All 15 patients demonstrate pressure relief)

Using outcomes data for marketing and business development begins with a close examination of outcomes achieved. Note findings:

### Outcome 1: Emergent care for wound infection, deteriorating wound status

A very important finding is that 94% of your patients did not require emergent care for wound infection or deterioration. One patient's environment was somewhat less than conducive for wound management. However, the patient did not want to leave her residence, and your agency agreed to work with her and the caretaker to meet the goal of allowing the patient to be cared for safely at her home. You discuss findings with the patient's physician and ask for guidance in the matter.

### Outcome 2: Increase in pressure ulcers

No patients had an increase in pressure ulcers. Both outcomes 1 and 2 provide powerful data for referral sources that are especially interested in cost containment. The number of urgent/emergent care visits and increase in the number of ulcers are two outcomes related to healthcare quality and costs.

### Outcome 3: Patient/caretaker demonstrates wound care management (i.e., dressing change, wound cleansing, infection control)

Eighty-six percent of your patients and/or caretakers perform wound management. This suggests that you are providing quality instruction, and also infers that you have been successful in teaching self-management skills, thus decreasing the need for additional urgent or emergent health services. Teaching a module of self-management skills can also be marketed as a program of special services.

While 86% is favorable, when you show that 86% of your patients/caretakers are independent with wound management, you leave your customer wondering about the remaining 14%. Be prepared to share your agency variance data and patient characteristics of this same group. Identify variances that may be affecting the remaining 14%. Look for lack of consistent caretaker, noncompliance, and difficulty with learning.

5

## CONCEPT APPLICATION:
### Using Outcomes Data for Marketing and Sales *(continued)*

*Outcome 4: Patient/caregiver verbalizes signs and symptoms of infection, wound deterioration and reports to homecare nurse/physician*

Ninety-three percent of your wound patients know the signs and symptoms of infection and wound deterioration. This indicates that your patients have the knowledge to facilitate early intervention if there are adverse signs or symptoms. This can also help decrease the need for urgent/emergent visits.

*Outcome 5: Patient/caretaker demonstrates proper pressure relief*

One hundred percent of patients/caretakers understand and demonstrate proper pressure relief. This helps to provide an appropriate surface for healing, and decreases the risk of wound deterioration, or the development of new wounds, which may directly affect re-hospitalization.

## AGENCY APPLICATION:
### Developing Outcome Indicators for Specific Customers

Identify **one** of your agency's **high volume referral sources**:

_____

Determine **one high-volume diagnosis** received from this referral source:

_____

Identify **one or two OASIS outcomes** pertinent to this diagnosis that the referral source may have interest in. Which OASIS outcomes have the potential of reflecting the quality of care or special services your agency delivers for this patient group?

_____

_____

Determine if other **agency supplemental outcomes** that this referral source wants his or her patients to achieve need to be measured. (Identify specific outcomes that the referral source is particularly interested in.) You may determine these from discussions with the referral source or in physician orders:

_____

_____

_____

_____

## AGENCY APPLICATION:

### Developing Outcome Indicators for Specific Customers
*(continued)*

Identify **best practice interventions** that are likely to have a positive effect on the outcomes identified:

_____

_____

_____

_____

_____

Identify **additional standards** of care that you would like to implement, based on an outcomes (process of care) investigation, chart review, and staff interviews:

_____

_____

_____

_____

Follow the outcomes for two or three quarters. Study your findings, paying particular attention to patient outcomes related to patient/caretaker self-management and compliance. Review financial outcomes to determine cost-effectiveness. Share outcomes with referral sources of choice. Enlist recommendations for further care enhancement.

Many homecare agencies tell their referral sources what they do and how well they do it. Few can actually demonstrate specific outcomes data for specific patient populations.

## POTENTIAL EFFECTS OF PATIENT OUTCOMES ON PHYSICIAN PRACTICE PATTERNS

Practice patterns can be defined as *interventions and general response tendencies of physicians* based on evidence and published data, experience and authority, as well as efficiency (Green, Gorenflo, and Wyszewianski, 2002). Sharing valid outcomes data with physicians and other referral sources can positively influence practice patterns that help achieve improved clinical and financial outcomes. Peer outcome information is helpful for a physician to use in light of outcomes data specific for his or her own patients (Baldwin, 2003).

Use your data to pinpoint quality of care issues when goals are not being met. Keep in mind there are times when a physician orders a specific number of visits for a patient and assumes that goals are achieved in this timeframe. Use your data to demonstrate how the patients are progressing and the timeframe in which outcomes are actually achieved.

For example, a surgeon typically orders SN 3wk1, 2wk1 for the instruction of stoma management for his patients with a new ostomy or those having complications, assuming that the patient will be able to manage in this timeframe. The clinicians do everything they can to discharge the patient within this frequency and duration, for he is a top referral source and is a very busy surgeon. Occasionally he is contacted for the approval of an additional visit, but as a rule, he consistently orders this frequency and duration.

The agency begins measuring the supplemental outcome, *Patient/caretaker independent with ostomy management at discharge*. For the past quarter, only 80% of this surgeon's patients achieve this outcome. By contrast, 98% of the patients of all other surgeons combined are discharged with independence in stoma management. However, the average number of visits for other patients with ostomy is eight. An agency manager meets with the surgeon whose patients are not achieving the better outcome. They discuss the elements of the agency's teaching module for the patient and caretaker. Outcomes data are shared, highlighting the comparison of the percentage of his patients with other surgeons as a whole.

The surgeon wants his patients to be independent at discharge, even though he has not articulated this clearly in his orders in the past. He recalls that two of his patients, during return follow-up office visits post homecare discharge, have expressed some anxiety in properly caring for the stoma. He decides to increase his frequency and duration to eight visits, thereby revising his previous practice pattern.

It is important to know that physicians differ measurably in what they consider credible sources of information, the weight they assign to practical concerns, and their willingness to diverge from group norms (Green et al., 2002). Knowing the patient outcomes of interest to them and having valid data to share is imperative. Ascertaining the type of patient outcomes that your referral sources are most interested in is an important first step.

Physician expectations for patients' clinical progress are often found in usual or *standing* home care orders. Other times, the physician may actually write or verbalize patient goals and/or expected results. This gives you outcomes to consider for measurement for that particular physician.

For example, an orthopedic surgeon has standing orders that include full weight bearing at discharge. This is an outcome of obvious importance to the surgeon and a supplemental outcome indicator that your agency can measure. Couple this outcome indicator with those related to the patient's compliance with the home exercise program and with the OASIS outcomes of function, and you have a well-rounded compliment of outcome measurements to share that are indicative of patient independence and progress.

## CONCEPT APPLICATION:
## Comparing Referral Source Outcomes Data

Benchmark the outcomes data of physicians or referral sources. Study the following example of comparative patient outcomes data for one physician as compared to a group of other physicians' patients.

**Table 5.1**  Comparative Outcomes Data

| Outcome Indicator | Physician X's patients | All other physician patients |
|---|---|---|
| Independent with stoma management at discharge | 1/6 | 5/5 |
| Average visits | 5 | 8 |
| Urgent office visits for complications | 3 | 0 |

## CONCEPT APPLICATION:
## Comparing Treatment Protocols

Physicians appreciate data that show actual differences in patient outcomes based on treatment protocols. The information is also helpful to the agency as it determines which physicians use evidence-based practice and clinical practice guidelines. Encourage these physicians to use your agency's services.

**Table 5.2**  Comparing Treatment Protocols

| Measurement | Physician X | Physician Y |
|---|---|---|
| Primary treatment | Wet-to-dry with saline | Advanced wound dressing |
| Avg. visits per episode | 120 | 24 |
| Avg. LOS | 4 episodes | 2 episodes |
| Total cost of care | $49,000 | $5,000 |

5

### AGENCY APPLICATION:
## Comparing Agency Treatment Protocols

Enter the following data for two of your agency's referral sources. Select one high-volume, primary diagnosis and compare treatment protocols, such as wound treatments or a special exercise program versus usual care. Compare applicable OASIS outcomes and pertinent agency supplemental outcomes, if available.

**Table 5.3** Comparing Agency Treatment Protocols

Primary Diagnosis: _____

| Measurement | Physician X | Physician Y |
|---|---|---|
| Outcome(s) of interest | | |
| Primary treatment | | |
| Avg. visits per episode | | |
| Avg. LOS | | |
| Total cost of care | $ | $ |

## EFFECT OF PATIENT OUTCOMES ON MCO DECISION MAKING

Managed care provides another opportunity for marketing your services according to outcomes achieved. Historically, the primary concerns of MCOs have been cost and resource utilization—choosing homecare services that support their cost containment strategies, while still providing an acceptable quality of care to their members (Weil, 2002). MCOs typically authorize a number of visits on admission. The agency must then achieve the results that can be realistically accomplished in this timeframe. In this way, MCOs dictate visit and discipline utilization.

However, valid outcomes data related to care quality, cost containment, and resource utilization can quantifiably demonstrate to the organization that the agency is interested in cost-effectiveness, and preserves and improves care quality. Providing clinical and financial outcomes data to the MCO verifies your interest and effectiveness as a partner in meeting mutual goals (Morrow, 2001). This can afford you a better position when negotiating contracts, as well as when discussing homecare needs for MCO member patients on a day-to-day basis.

Sharing desired outcomes achieved can also set the stage for a trusting relationship to emerge. MCOs have a vested interest in agency outcomes that reveal an improvement in LOS, visit utilization, decreased acute care readmissions, and the need for urgent/emergent care, all of which carry a high price tag for third-party payers.

## PREPARING OUTCOMES PRESENTATIONS FOR CUSTOMERS

Consider eliciting feedback from your customers regarding the format they find the most reader-friendly, and at what intervals they wish to receive data. The following are important considerations for planning and presenting outcome-based presentations for customers:

## Planning

- Time allotted by the customer for the presentation.
- The most appropriate visual aid(s) for the setting, such as Microsoft® PowerPoint for larger groups, a flip chart for singles or groups of five or less, or pamphlets or brochures when a personal presentation of data is not an option.
- Selecting a format that is professional, streamlined, and easy to review.
- Prioritizing critical information for a particular customer.
- Providing valid outcomes data for review.

## Presentation

- The introduction
- Outcomes of primary interest to the customer
- Outcomes that you feel show a tremendous improvement in quality and cost-effectiveness over a recent period of time
- Outcomes of specialty programs or new services
- The format that demonstrates the best visual of outcomes achieved, such as bar graphs, pie charts, or run charts
- Data comparison of patient outcomes before and after implementation of specific best practice interventions
- Correlation of clinical and financial outcomes specific to treatment modalities
- Characteristics of customer's patient population(s) compared with others

### Guiding Questions

- Have you focused the presentation on outcomes particular to the customer?
- Who will be aggregating outcomes data and verifying their accuracy for the presentation?
- At what intervals will data be aggregated for presentation to your customers?
- Who will present the data to your customers?
- Who will prepare the data in a professional format?

### REFERENCES

Baldwin, H. (2003, April). Integrity drives productivity. *Selling Power Magazine*, 70–72.

Bly, R. W. (2003, February). Fool proof marketing. *Home Business Magazine*, 218.

Dinsdale, S. J. & Taylor, J. (2003). The value of loyalty. *Optimize Magazine*, issue 18. Retrieved September 30, 2003 from http://www.optimizemag.com/issue/018/marketing, htm.

Green, A. G., Gorenflo, D. W., & Wyszewianski, L. (2002). Validating an instrument for selecting interventions to change physician practice patterns: A Michigan consortium for family practice research study. *Journal of Family Practice*, 51(11), 938. Retrieved October 6, 2003 from Infotrac database.

Hill, M. (1999). Outcomes measurements require nursing to shift to outcome-based practice. *Nursing Administration Quarterly*, 24(1), 1–9. Retrieved January 8, 2003 from Infotrac database.

Lapin, L. M. (2001). Data management: Strategies to bridge financial and clinical information. *Remington Report*, 9(6), 34.

Morrow, T. (2001, March). New opportunities for an old disease. Presented at the Dupont Pharmaceuticals Advisory Board for Innohep, Chicago, Illinois.

Potts, J. (2001). Thriving under PPS: How to harness the power of data. *Remington Report*, 9(3), 76–77.

Ratner, E. (2002a). Physicians as key customers in home care. *Remington Report*, 10(4), 36; 38.

Ratner, E. (2002b). Reluctant partnership or blissful marriage: The home health agency and doctor relationship. *Remington Report*, 10(6), 32.

Rich, P. J. & Davis, G. S. (2002, Fall). Tiered benefit HMO plans: The next generation of managed care plans. *Managed Care Quarterly*, 54–59.

Rooney, H. & Lang, C. (2003). Key performance measures. *Remington Report*, 11(1), 14; 16–18.

Sblendorio, S. (2003). From data overload to information management and decision support. *Remington Report*, 11(2), 5–8.

Weil, T. P. (2002). Managed competition using both market driven and regulatory strategies. *Managed Care Quarterly*, 10(3), 32.

Wincel, J. (2002, August). Competitive partnerships. *Optimize Magazine*, Issue 10. Retrieved September 30, 2003 from http://www.optimizemag.com/issue/010/collaborative. htm.

5

# Appendices

Agency for Healthcare Research and Quality
www.ahrq.gov

American Academy of Neurology
www.aan.com/professionals/practice/guidelines.cfm

American Academy of Pediatrics
www.aap.org/policy/paramtoc.html

American Academy of Physical Medicine and
Rehabilitation
aapmr.org/hpl/pracguide/resources/htm

American College of Cardiology
www.acc.org/clinical/statements.htm

American College of Physicians
www.acponline.org/sci-policy/guidelines

American Diabetes Association
www.diabetes.org

American Dietetic Association
www.eatright.org

American Heart Association
www.aha.org

American Liver Foundation
www.liverfoundation.org

American Lung Association
www.lungusa.org

American Psychiatric Association
www.psych.org/clin__res/prac_guide.cfm

Centers for Disease Control
www.cdc.gov

Center for Evidence-Based Medicine
www.cebm.jr.ox.ac.uk

Cochrane Collaboration, The
www.cochrane.org

Delmarva Foundation for Medical Care
www.homehealth.dfmc.org

Disease Management Association of America
www.aishealth.com/products

Evidence-Based Medicine Resources
www.ebmny.org/cpg.html

Evidenced-Based Nursing
www.ebn.bmjjournals.com

Healthcare Corporate Compliance Center
www.corpcompliance.com

Infectious Disease Society of America
www.idsociety.org/pg/toc.htm

National Institute of Diabetes
www.niddk.nih.gov

National Guidelines Clearinghouse
www.nhlbi.nih.gov/guidelines
www.guideline.gov

National Institute on Aging
www.nia.nih.gov

National Institutes of Health
www.nlm.nih.gov

National Institutes of Health—Healthstat
www.hstat.nlm.nih.gov/hq/Hquest/screen/HquestHome

National Library of Medicine
www.pubmed.com

Occupational Safety and Health Administration
www.osha.gov

Prevention Guidelines System, The
www.phppo.cdc.gov/CDCRecommends/AdvSearchV.asp

Primary Care Clinical Practice Guidelines
www.medicine.ucsf.edu/resources/guidelines

Selected Evidence-Based Healthcare Resources
www.health.library.mcgill.ca/resources/ebmlist.htm

User's Guide to Medical Literature
www.health.library.mcgill.ca/resource/userguides.htm

U.S. National Heart, Lung and Blood Institute
www.nhlbi.nih.gov

Wound, Ostomy, Continence Nurses Society
www.wocn.org

# Action Plan: OBQI/OBQM

| Category | Action Items | Completion Date | Responsible Person(s) | Methods |
|---|---|---|---|---|
| *(Subjects to be addressed)* | *(Action to be taken through discussion and evaluation, recommendation, assessment, and education)* | *Target date for completion of action items* | *Person(s) assigned to tasks* | *Method(s) used* |
| 1. Designation of OASIS leadership roles (can be one or more persons) | 1. Ensure accuracy of responses to OASIS data set items and accuracy of data entry. <br> 2. Coordinate and facilitate OASIS outcomes evaluation, interpretation, and analyses. <br> 3. Coordinate focus group or PI team efforts for outcomes investigation and recommendations for improvement or remediation. <br> 4. Coordinate involvement of all levels of clinical staff. | | | |
| 2. Verification of OASIS data accuracy | 1. Staff use of proper response instructions for OASIS data set items: <br> • Orientation and annual retraining <br> • Annual OASIS competency <br> • Annual performance evaluation <br> 2. Clinical record review. <br> 3. Quarterly, clinical OASIS onsite visit audits. | | | |
| 3. OASIS Data Processing & Transmission | 1. Timeliness of data transmission. <br> 2. Accuracy of OASIS clinical data entry. (Monthly data entry audit) <br> 3. Review of Final Validation Report. | | | |

## Action Plan: OBQI/OBQM

| Category | Action Items | Completion Date | Responsible Person(s) | Methods |
|---|---|---|---|---|
| 4. Analyses of OASIS Outcome Reports | 1. Review of Case Mix Profile Report during same time period of OASIS outcome reports.<br>2. Overall review of OASIS Outcome Reports. | | | |
| 5. Selection of Target Outcomes | 1. Selection made one–two weeks after report becomes available.<br>2. Use of OBQI criteria for selection of *target* outcome(s):<br>• Statistically significant differences between agency outcomes and national reference (indicated on the report as * or ** or + or ++)<br>• Larger magnitude of the difference in outcome percentages<br>• At least 30 cases<br>• Level of significance at or less than .10. If none, those closest to .10, but not greater than .25.<br>• Relevance to agency goals or PI initiatives<br>• Relevance to clinical quality of care<br>3. Use of OBQM criteria for selection of *priority* outcome(s):<br>• Review the Case Mix Profile report in depth.<br>• Note those areas having asterisks of significance, but do not limit to these alone.<br>• Review Adverse Event Outcomes Report.<br>• Of these, select those that have the greatest relevance to your patient populations. | | | |

**Action Plan: OBQI/OBQM**

| Category | Action Items | Completion Date | Responsible Person(s) | Methods |
|---|---|---|---|---|
| 6. Outcomes Investigation | 1. Identify the aspects of care that *should be* provided related to the outcome.<br>2. Outline the care actually provided.<br>3. Use this outline for chart review.<br>4. Aggregate findings.<br>5. Summarize conclusions. | | | |
| 7. Plan and Implementation to Improve Care | 1. Write Clear Statement(s) of Problem or Strength.<br>2. Identify specific actions (best practices) intended to improve the target outcome.<br>3. Determine resources needed to implement best practices (i.e., man, machine, tools, process).<br>4. Outline components of staff education/competency.<br>5. Schedule and conduct staff education/competency.<br>6. Schedule the date of implementation of best practice (OBQI recommends within one month of obtaining report). | | | |
| 8. Implementation Follow-up | Perform follow-up within two–three weeks of implementation:<br>• Feedback from staff<br>• Sample chart review<br>• Review OBQI / OBQM outcome reports at the next quarter to determine if improvement has occurred<br>• Communicate follow-up findings to staff<br>• Reinforce acceptable outcomes | | | |

## Action Plan: Care Pathways

| Category | Action Items | Completion Date | Responsible Person(s) | Methods |
|---|---|---|---|---|
| *Major categories to be addressed* | *Elements to be addressed through discussion and evaluation, recommendation, assessment, and education* | *Date for completion of action items* | *Person(s) for assigned tasks* | *Method(s) used* |
| 1. Designation of leadership roles | 1. Evaluation of resources<br>2. Timeline approval for pathway implementation<br>3. Pathway development<br>4. Staff education<br>5. Staff competency assessment<br>6. Pathway implementation | | | |
| 2. Evaluation of Resources | **Human Resources**<br>Evaluate agency experience for pathway development<br>Contract consulting versus in-house<br><br>**Financial Resources**<br>1. Evaluate type of pathways most suited:<br> • IS ability to develop in-house software and related needs.<br> • Purchase of software and point-of-care device.<br> • Purchase of manually documented pathways.<br> • Scanning technology & manual pathways.<br>2. Determine cost of contract versus in-house development.<br>3. Cost of developing versus purchase of patient teaching materials. | | | |
| 3. Develop timeline for implementation | Complete action plan for leadership approval. | | | |

## Action Plan: Care Pathways

| Category | Action Items | Completion Date | Responsible Person(s) | Methods |
|---|---|---|---|---|
| 4. Pathway Development | 1. Prioritize pathways for development:<br> • Identify primary patient populations<br> • Evaluate staff experience and expertise for populations served<br> • Identify OASIS target outcomes that a pathway could potentially improve | | | |
| a. Develop a format | 1. Define the categories of care that are pertinent to your overall populations.<br>2. Select a style. | | | |
| b. Research best practice for diagnoses, conditions, or procedures selected | 1. Review the literature at the library or access the Internet.<br>2. Review agency standards of care, and policy and procedure that exists relative to the literature.<br>3. Compile best practice interventions for each pathway. | | | |
| c. Conduct a medical record review | 1. Specify the audit tool to be used.<br>2. Outline physician practice patterns.<br>3. Note patient teaching materials used by staff.<br>4. Note clinician interventions for all disciplines.<br>5. Note intervention overlap by disciplines. | | | |
| d. Evaluate current agency teaching materials for pathway use | 1. Compare current material content to literature best practice.<br>2. Determine if revisions to agency materials are needed.<br>3. Evaluate purchase versus in-house development.<br>4. Determine how to organize patient teaching materials for easy staff access.<br>5. Outline process for staff to obtain teaching materials.<br>6. Identify who will maintain patient teaching materials. | | | |

**Action Plan: Care Pathways**

| Category | Action Items | Completion Date | Responsible Person(s) | Methods |
|---|---|---|---|---|
| e. Determine if changes are needed to product lines or supplies | 1. Identify and evaluate supplies and products.<br>2. Make recommendations for change if needed.<br>3. Determine the financial impact of recommendations. | | | |
| f. Identify outcomes for each pathway | 1. Establish a set of outcomes for each pathway that corresponds with interventions provided.<br>2. Determine frequency of outcomes aggregation and analyses. | | | |
| g. Determine number of visits appropriate for each discipline for each pathway | 1. Review the agency's current average number of visits for each discipline for the diagnosis in question.<br>2. Assign the number of visits needed to help achieve the desired outcome in a cost-efficient manner. | | | |
| h. Evaluate the need for new or additional staff competencies | 1. Compare existing competency requirements with those required by best practice.<br>2. Identify those required for each discipline as needed.<br>3. Determine how the competency can best be assessed.<br>4. Choose a timeframe for assessing the competency. | | | |
| i. Identify variances | 1. List variances to be tracked.<br>2. Determine how and when these are to be reported by staff.<br>3. Determine method of aggregation.<br>4. Select the frequency of variance aggregation and analyses. | | | |
| 5. Staff Education | 1. Outline agency content for all disciplines.<br>2. Determine times and locations.<br>3. Discuss issues for weekend and evening staff.<br>4. Determine teaching methods.<br>5. Develop materials. | | | |

# Action Plan: Care Pathways

| Category | Action Items | Completion Date | Responsible Person(s) | Methods |
|---|---|---|---|---|
| 6. Staff Competency | 1. Determine need for new or changed competencies.<br>2. Identify which staff are affected.<br>3. Identify best method to involve contract staff, as needed.<br>4. Outline process for competency assessment.<br>5. Determine times and locations. | | | |
| 7. Pathway Implementation | 1. Finalize process for pathway use.<br>2. Decide how many pathways to implement initially.<br>3. Set dates for implementation.<br>4. Identify facilitators of the implementation process for staff.<br>5. Plan first formal 3–4 week follow-up.<br> • Conduct clinical documentation reviews to determine accuracy of outcome measurement and timeliness of initiation of pathway and implementation of appropriate interventions.<br> • Obtain feedback from all staff.<br> • Solicit input for revision of process, pathway content, and teaching materials.<br>6. Plan for revisions. | | | |

## Action Plan: DM

| Category | Action Items | Completion Date | Responsible Person(s) | Methods |
|---|---|---|---|---|
| *Major Planning* | *Elements to be addressed through discussion and evaluation, recommendation, assessment, and education* | *Date for completion of action items* | *Person(s) for assigned tasks* | *Method(s) used* |
| 1. Agency Preparedness for DM | 1. Selection of care pathway format and method.<br>2. Selection of individual to coordinate DM efforts.<br>3. Selection of individual to coordinate marketing efforts. | | | |
| 2. Prioritization of DM Diagnoses for Agency Implementation | 1. Identify primary patient populations by:<br>• Diagnosis<br>• Volume<br>• Demographics<br>• Referral sources<br>• Co-morbidities<br>• Preventative measures<br>2. Specify the populations that have greatest potential for improvement in clinical outcomes.<br>3. Determine the existence of DM initiatives by hospitals and clinics in your area, as well as MCOs for whom clients your agency is providing care.<br>4. Contact these providers to determine their interest in forming a DM continuum. | | | |
| 3. Use of Evidence-based Guidelines for Care Pathway Interventions | 1. Research valid health literature for evidence-based interventions.<br>2. Evaluate the relevance of each intervention to intended agency patient populations. | | | |

## Action Plan: DM

| Category | Action Items | Completion Date | Responsible Person(s) | Methods |
|---|---|---|---|---|
| 3. Use of Evidence-based Guidelines for Care Pathway Interventions *(continued)* | 3. Formulate interventions for each DM diagnosis.<br>4. Determine disciplines that provide care and the number of visits planned.<br>5. Enter these into your agency's care pathway format.<br>6. Include supplies and product lines that are affected by interventions.<br>7. Evaluate financial impact of interventions. | | | |
| 4. Patient/Caretaker Self-Management Education | 1. Select or develop patient/caretaker teaching materials for the DM care pathway(s).<br>2. Discuss appropriateness of home care as the vehicle for teaching:<br>• Primary prevention and risk assessment<br>• Behavior modification techniques<br>• Compliance/surveillance<br>3. Discuss need for training clinicians to teach patient/caretaker self-management.<br>4. Determine the type of patient support and surveillance needed. | | | |
| 5. Collaboration with Referral Sources and Support Service Providers | 1. Contact referral sources to determine support of DM interventions and mission.<br>2. Contact DME providers to determine interest and ability to efficiently provide supplies and equipment. | | | |

## Action Plan: DM

| Category | Action Items | Completion Date | Responsible Person(s) | Methods |
|---|---|---|---|---|
| 6. Outcome Measurement and Evaluation | 1. Select OASIS outcomes and agency outcomes for each DM diagnosis, according to interventions provided.<br>2. Determine causes of variance that will be aggregated.<br>3. Determine frequency of outcome and variance aggregation and analyses. | | | |
| 7. Routine Reporting and Feedback Loop | 1. Identify providers and individuals in the feedback loop.<br>2. Determine the feedback mechanism and the type of information to be shared. | | | |
| 8. Development of DM Marketing Plan | 1. Note key referral sources in the agency's feedback loop.<br>2. Select appropriate method of providing patient outcomes data for referral sources. | | | |
| 9. Annual Agency Evaluation | 1. Prepare OASIS and agency supplemental patient outcomes data for presentation and discussion.<br>2. Prepare to discuss staff competency and competency assessment needs relative to outcomes desired and outcomes achieved. | | | |

**Illness/Condition:** _____

**Literature Search Resource(s):** _____

**Performed by:** _____  **Date:** _____

| Assessments (Specify: patient risk, pain, home, safety, other) |
| --- |
| |
| **Diagnostic Tests** |
| 1. |
| 2. |
| 3. |
| **Medications** |
| |
| **Nutrition/Hydration** |
| 1. |
| 2. |
| 3. |
| 4. |
| **Mobility/Rehabilitation** |
| 1. |
| 2. |
| 3. |
| 4. |
| 5. |
| **Home Equipment** |
| 1. |
| 2. |
| 3. |
| **Psychosocial** |
| 1. |
| 2. |
| 3. |
| **Self-Management Skills** |
| 1. |
| 2. |
| 3. |
| 4. |
| 5. |
| 6. |
| 7. |

**Agency:** _____

**Illness/Condition:** _____  **Performed by:** _____  **Date:** _____

| Medical Record | 1 | 2 | 3 | 4 | 5 | 6 | 7 | 8 | 9 | 10 |
|---|---|---|---|---|---|---|---|---|---|---|
| **Record Identifier** | | | | | | | | | | |
| **Category/Interventions** | | | | | | | | | | |
| *Assessment (patient risk, pain, home, safety, med)* | | | | | | | | | | |
|    RN | | | | | | | | | | |
|    PT / OT / SLP (circle) | | | | | | | | | | |
|    Other | | | | | | | | | | |
| *Disease Process & Adverse S / S* | | | | | | | | | | |
| | | | | | | | | | | |
| *Diagnostic Tests (types)* | | | | | | | | | | |
| 1. | | | | | | | | | | |
| 2. | | | | | | | | | | |
| 3. | | | | | | | | | | |
| *Medications* | | | | | | | | | | |
| | | | | | | | | | | |
| *Nutrition/Hydration (specify)* | | | | | | | | | | |
| 1. | | | | | | | | | | |
| 2. | | | | | | | | | | |
| 3. | | | | | | | | | | |
| 4. | | | | | | | | | | |
| *Mobility/Rehabilitation (specify tx)* | | | | | | | | | | |
| 1. | | | | | | | | | | |
| 2. | | | | | | | | | | |
| 3. | | | | | | | | | | |
| 4. | | | | | | | | | | |
| 5. | | | | | | | | | | |
| *Home Equipment (types used)* | | | | | | | | | | |
| 1. | | | | | | | | | | |
| 2. | | | | | | | | | | |
| 3. | | | | | | | | | | |
| *Psychosocial (issues addressed)* | | | | | | | | | | |
| 1. | | | | | | | | | | |
| 2. | | | | | | | | | | |
| 3. | | | | | | | | | | |
| *Self-Management Skills (specify)* | | | | | | | | | | |
| 1. | | | | | | | | | | |
| 2. | | | | | | | | | | |
| 3. | | | | | | | | | | |
| 4. | | | | | | | | | | |
| 5. | | | | | | | | | | |
| 6. | | | | | | | | | | |
| 7. | | | | | | | | | | |

**Pathway:** _____

|  | SN | Therapy | HHA | Other |
|---|---|---|---|---|
| Assessments | _____ | _____ | _____ | _____ |
| Diagnostics | _____ | _____ | | |
| | _____ | _____ | | |
| Procedures | _____ | _____ | _____ | |
| Disease Process | _____ | _____ | | _____ |
| Medications | _____ | _____ | | |
| Nutrition/ Hydration | _____ | | _____ | |
| | _____ | | _____ | _____ |
| | _____ | | _____ | |
| | _____ | | | |
| Mobility/ Rehabilitation | _____ | _____ | _____ | |
| | _____ | _____ | _____ | |
| | | _____ | | |
| | | _____ | | |
| Safe/Proper Use Equipment | _____ | _____ | | |
| | _____ | _____ | | |
| Psychosocial | _____ | _____ | | |
| Self-Mgt Skills | _____ | _____ | | |
| | _____ | _____ | | |
| | _____ | _____ | | |
| | _____ | _____ | | |

*Instructions:* Enter discipline abbrev. in the boxes that correspond to planned visit interventions over the course of an episode. Enter # of Disciplines per day and Visits per week at the bottom.
*Key:* **N**: Nurse / **Ps**: Psyche / **A**: Aide / **P**: Physical Therapist / **O**: Occupational Therapist / **S**: Speech Therapist / **D**: Dietitian / **SS**: Social Service / Other _____: _____

**Care Pathway Name:**_____  **Wk # (     )**          **Wk # (     )**

| Enter agency's Medicare weekdays | | | | | | | | | | | | | | | |
|---|---|---|---|---|---|---|---|---|---|---|---|---|---|---|---|
| *Interventions* | *Planned Visits* | | | | | | | | | | | | | | |
| **Disease Process/Adverse S&S** | | | | | | | | | | | | | | | |
| **Diagnostics/Procedures** | | | | | | | | | | | | | | | |
| 1. | | | | | | | | | | | | | | | |
| 2. | | | | | | | | | | | | | | | |
| 3. | | | | | | | | | | | | | | | |
| **Medications** | | | | | | | | | | | | | | | |
| **Nutrition/Hydration** | | | | | | | | | | | | | | | |
| 1. | | | | | | | | | | | | | | | |
| 2. | | | | | | | | | | | | | | | |
| 3. | | | | | | | | | | | | | | | |
| 4. | | | | | | | | | | | | | | | |
| **Mobility/Rehabilitation** | | | | | | | | | | | | | | | |
| 1. | | | | | | | | | | | | | | | |
| 2. | | | | | | | | | | | | | | | |
| 3. | | | | | | | | | | | | | | | |
| 4. | | | | | | | | | | | | | | | |
| 5. | | | | | | | | | | | | | | | |
| **Home Equipment** | | | | | | | | | | | | | | | |
| 1. | | | | | | | | | | | | | | | |
| 2. | | | | | | | | | | | | | | | |
| 3. | | | | | | | | | | | | | | | |
| **Psychosocial** | | | | | | | | | | | | | | | |
| 1. | | | | | | | | | | | | | | | |
| 2. | | | | | | | | | | | | | | | |
| 3. | | | | | | | | | | | | | | | |
| 4. | | | | | | | | | | | | | | | |
| 5. | | | | | | | | | | | | | | | |
| **Self-Management Skills** | | | | | | | | | | | | | | | |
| 1. | | | | | | | | | | | | | | | |
| 2. | | | | | | | | | | | | | | | |
| 3. | | | | | | | | | | | | | | | |
| 4. | | | | | | | | | | | | | | | |
| 5. | | | | | | | | | | | | | | | |

| # of Disciplines per Day | | | | | | | | | | | | | | |
|---|---|---|---|---|---|---|---|---|---|---|---|---|---|---|
| **Total Visits: per Week / per Episode** | | | | / | | | | | | / | | | |

**Pathway:** _____

**Topic:** _____   **Information:** _____

**Pathway:** _____

**Write the outcome indicator, its measurement timeframe, and who will measure.**

1. _____

2. _____

3. _____

4. _____

5. _____

6. _____

7. _____

8. _____

9. _____

10. _____

11. _____

12. _____

13. _____

14. _____

15. _____

**Agency:** _____

**Care Pathway:** _____

**Monthly / Quarterly**

**Date:** _____   **Number of Patients (N): :** _____

| Outcome Indicators<br>(Abbreviate by subject matter) | # Met / # Appl = % Met | | | # Not / # Appl = % Not<br>Met | | | # NA / Total N = % NA | | |
|---|---|---|---|---|---|---|---|---|---|
| 1. | | | | | | | | | |
| 2. | | | | | | | | | |
| 3. | | | | | | | | | |
| 4. | | | | | | | | | |
| 5. | | | | | | | | | |
| 6. | | | | | | | | | |
| 7. | | | | | | | | | |
| 8. | | | | | | | | | |
| 9. | | | | | | | | | |
| 10. | | | | | | | | | |
| 11. | | | | | | | | | |
| 12. | | | | | | | | | |
| 13. | | | | | | | | | |
| 14. | | | | | | | | | |
| 15. | | | | | | | | | |

**User's Key:**

**# Met:** Number of patients who met the outcome; **% Met:** Percentage of patients who met the outcome.

**# Not Met:** Number of patients who did not meet the outcome; **% Not Met:** Percentage of patients who did not meet the outcome.

**# Appl:** Total number of patients for whom the outcome applies; (# Met + the # Not Met).

**# NA:** Total number of patients for whom the outcome is not applicable; **% NA:** Percent of patient group for whom the outcome is not applicable.

**Total N=** Total number of patients in the group.

# Outcomes Trending Report (Monthly)

Agency: _____

Q _____ / Year: _____

Pathway: _____

| Outcome Indicators | Month _____ %Met | %Not Met | %NA | Month _____ %Met | %Not Met | %NA | Month _____ %Met | %Not Met | %NA |
|---|---|---|---|---|---|---|---|---|---|
| 1. | | | | | | | | | |
| 2. | | | | | | | | | |
| 3. | | | | | | | | | |
| 4. | | | | | | | | | |
| 5. | | | | | | | | | |
| 6. | | | | | | | | | |
| 7. | | | | | | | | | |
| 8. | | | | | | | | | |
| 9. | | | | | | | | | |
| 10. | | | | | | | | | |
| 11. | | | | | | | | | |
| 12. | | | | | | | | | |
| 13. | | | | | | | | | |
| 14. | | | | | | | | | |
| 15. | | | | | | | | | |

# Outcomes Trending Report (Quarterly)

**Agency:** _____

**Year:** _____

**Pathway:** _____

| Outcome Indicators | Quarters | % Met | | | | | | | | % Not Met | | | | | | | | % NA | | | |
|---|---|---|---|---|---|---|---|---|---|---|---|---|---|---|---|---|---|---|---|---|---|
| | | Q1 | Q2 | Q3 | Q4 | | | | | Q1 | Q2 | Q3 | Q4 | | | | | Q1 | Q2 | Q3 | Q4 |
| 1. | | | | | | | | | | | | | | | | | | | | | |
| 2. | | | | | | | | | | | | | | | | | | | | | |
| 3. | | | | | | | | | | | | | | | | | | | | | |
| 4. | | | | | | | | | | | | | | | | | | | | | |
| 5. | | | | | | | | | | | | | | | | | | | | | |
| 6. | | | | | | | | | | | | | | | | | | | | | |
| 7. | | | | | | | | | | | | | | | | | | | | | |
| 8. | | | | | | | | | | | | | | | | | | | | | |
| 9. | | | | | | | | | | | | | | | | | | | | | |
| 10. | | | | | | | | | | | | | | | | | | | | | |
| 11. | | | | | | | | | | | | | | | | | | | | | |
| 12. | | | | | | | | | | | | | | | | | | | | | |
| 13. | | | | | | | | | | | | | | | | | | | | | |
| 14. | | | | | | | | | | | | | | | | | | | | | |
| 15. | | | | | | | | | | | | | | | | | | | | | |

**Agency:** _____

**Date:** _____

| Descriptors | High Risk | High Volume | Correlates with critical outcome | Lack of knowledge | Other | Non-essential |
|---|---|---|---|---|---|---|
| **Best Practice Interventions** | | | | | | |
| 1. | | | | | | |
| 2. | | | | | | |
| 3. | | | | | | |
| 4. | | | | | | |
| 5. | | | | | | |
| 6. | | | | | | |
| 7. | | | | | | |
| 8. | | | | | | |
| 9. | | | | | | |
| 10. | | | | | | |
| 11. | | | | | | |
| 12. | | | | | | |
| 13. | | | | | | |
| 14. | | | | | | |
| 15. | | | | | | |
| 16. | | | | | | |
| 17. | | | | | | |
| 18. | | | | | | |
| 19. | | | | | | |
| 20. | | | | | | |

**Employee Name/Title:** _____

**Full T / Part T / PRN / Wkend / Contract**

| Competency Indicator | S | U | Date | (R) | (R) D | Comments | Signature(s) |
|---|---|---|---|---|---|---|---|
| | | | | | | | |
| | | | | | | | |
| | | | | | | | |
| | | | | | | | |
| | | | | | | | |
| | | | | | | | |
| | | | | | | | |
| | | | | | | | |
| | | | | | | | |
| | | | | | | | |
| | | | | | | | |
| | | | | | | | |
| | | | | | | | |
| | | | | | | | |
| | | | | | | | |
| | | | | | | | |
| | | | | | | | |
| | | | | | | | |

**User's Key:**

**S:** Satisfactory *(may enter numerical score)*
**U:** Unsatisfactory *(may enter numerical score)*
**Date:** Date competency assessed
**(R):** Remediation required *(indicate by checkmark)*
**(R)D:** Date of remediation
**Comments:** *(may continue on back)*
**Signature:** Assessor's Validation Signature

# Subject Index

# *Notes*